AF365862

SRI AUROBINDO AND MOTHER

FINDING THE PSYCHIC BEING

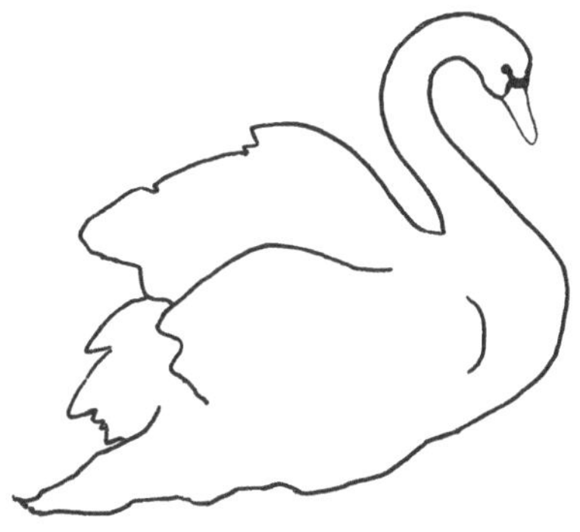

Impressum

Acknowledgments: This book contains quotations from Sri Aurobindo and Mother which were used in an exhibition titled "Sri Aurobindo and Mother, Finding the Psychic Being". In the yoga of personal growth and transformation which Sri Aurobindo and the Mother brought to humanity, the first stage to be attained is the realization of the individual soul, termed the "Psychic Being".

First Edition 2012
Second Editon 2022
Finding the Psychic Being
Loretta Shartsis

© The copyright holder for The Mother's Agenda is "Institut de Recherches Evolutives".

All rights reserved. No part of this book may be reprinted or reproduced or utilized in any form or by any electronic, mechanical, or other means, now known or hereafter invented, including photocopying and recording, or in any information storage or retrieval system, without permission in writing from the publishers.

ISBN 978-81-957301-8-6 (print)
ISBN 978-81-957301-9-3 (ebook)

BISAC Code:
OCC000000, BODY, MIND & SPIRIT / General
HEA025000, HEALTH & FITNESS / Yoga
REF019000, REFERENCE / Quotations

Thema Subject Category:
QD, Philosophy
VX, Mind, body, spirit

Cataloging-in-Publication Data for this title is available from the Library of Congress.

Printed and bound in India by:
PRISMA, Aurelec/ Prayogshala,
Auroville 605101, Tamil Nadu, India

Digital Editions produced by:
DMI Systems Pvt Ltd, Vishnupuri,
Aligarh 202001, Uttar Pradesh, India

Published by PRISMA, an imprint of Digital Media Initiatives
www.prisma.haus, www.dmi.systems

INTRODUCTION

This book contains quotations from Sri Aurobindo and Mother which were used in an exhibition titled "Sri Aurobindo and Mother, Finding the Psychic Being". In the yoga of personal growth and transformation which Sri Aurobindo and the Mother brought to humanity, the first stage to be attained is the realization of the individual soul, termed the "Psychic Being".

In Sri Aurobindo's epic poem, "Savitri", two people take inner journeys to find their psychic being. The exhibition was presented in the form of a journey which we all can take to find our own psychic being. This book contains the quotations in the order they were given in the exhibition so the reader can take the journey.

The quotations come from a variety of sources. Quotations from Sri Aurobindo are identified by his symbol and Quotations from Mother are identified by her symbol . References listing the actual sources can be found at the end of the book.

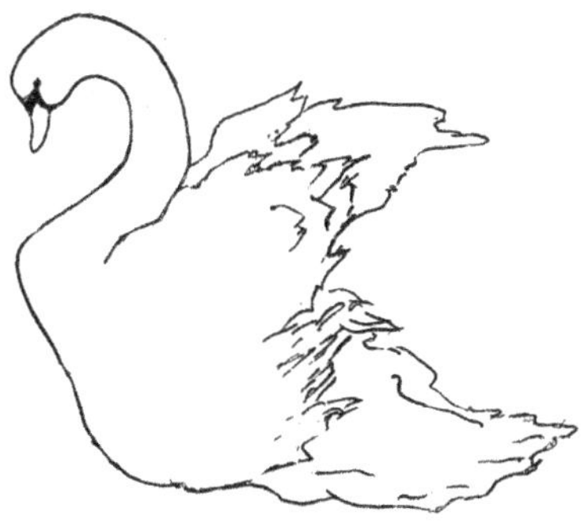

The Swan is the Indian symbol of the individual soul, the central being, the divine part which is turned towards the Divine, descending from there and ascending to it.

SOUL IN THE IGNORANCE

Soul in the Ignorance, wake from its stupor.
Flake of the world-fire, spark of Divinity.
Lift up thy mind and thy heart into glory.
Sun in the darkness, recover thy luster.

One, universal, ensphering creation,
Wheeling no more with inconscient Nature,
Feel thyself God-born, know thyself deathless.
Timeless return to thy immortal existence.

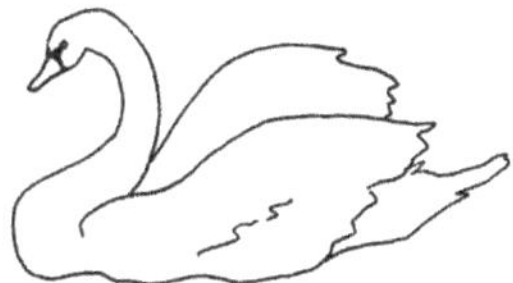

*What exactly is the soul or psychic being? And what is
meant by the evolution of the psychic being? What is its
relation to the Supreme?*

The soul and the psychic being are not exactly the same thing,
although their essence is the same.

The soul is the divine spark that dwells at the centre of
each being; it is identical with its Divine Origin; it is the divine
in man.

The psychic being is formed progressively around this
divine centre, the soul, in the course of its innumerable lives
in the terrestrial evolution, until the time comes when the
psychic being, fully formed and wholly awakened, becomes
the conscious sheath of the soul around which it is formed.

And thus identified with the Divine, it becomes His perfect
instrument in the world.

There is a nirvana behind the vital, a nirvana behind the psychic, a nirvana behind the mind; there is a nirvana on every level, even behind the physical - it's death. And those who withdraw, who try to attain Nirvana, NEVER go into the psychic - the psychic is something essentially linked to divine manifestation, not to divine non-intervention, not to Nirvana.

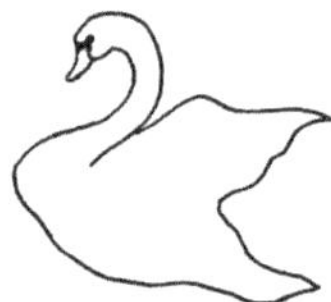

Earth must transform herself and equal Heaven
Or Heaven descend into earth's mortal state.
But for such vast spiritual change to be,
Out of the mystic cavern in man's heart
The heavenly Psyche must put off her veil
And step into common nature's crowded rooms
And stand uncovered in that nature's front
And rule its thoughts and fill the body and life.   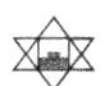

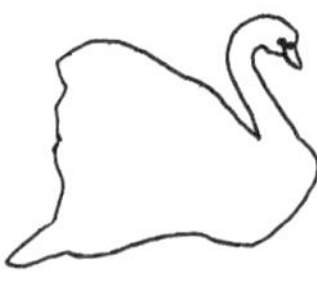

It is necessary to understand clearly the difference between the evolving soul (psychic being) and the pure Atman, self or spirit. The pure self is unborn, does not pass through death or birth, is independent of birth or body, mind or life or this manifested Nature. It is not bound by these things, not limited, not affected, even though it assumes and supports them. The soul, on the contrary, is something that comes down into birth and passes through death — although it does not itself die, for it is immortal — from one state to another, from the earth plane to other planes and back again to the earth-existence. It goes on with this progression from life to life through an evolution which leads it up to the human state and evolves through it all a being of itself which we call the psychic being that supports the evolution and develops a physical, a vital, a mental human consciousness as its instruments of world-experience and of a disguised, imperfect, but growing self-expression. All this it does from behind a veil showing something of its divine self only in so far as the imperfection of the instrumental being will allow it. But a time comes when it is able to prepare to come out from behind the veil, to take command and turn all the instrumental nature towards a divine fulfillment. This is the beginning of the true spiritual life. The soul is able now to make itself ready for a higher evolution of manifested consciousness than the mental human — it can pass from the mental to the spiritual and through degrees of the spiritual to the supramental state. Till then there is no reason why it should cease from birth, it cannot in fact do so. If having reached the spiritual state, it wills to pass out of the terrestrial manifestation, it may indeed do so — but there is also possible a higher manifestation, in the Knowledge and not in the Ignorance.

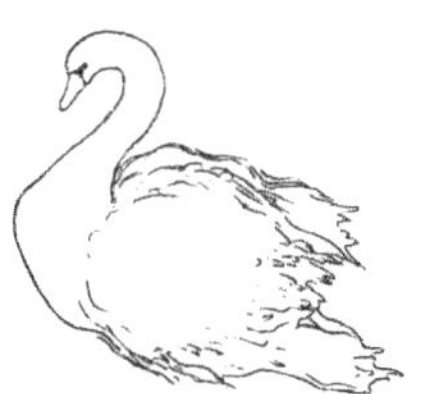

Hid deep in man celestial powers can dwell.
His fragile ship conveys through the sea of years
An incognito of the Imperishable.
A spirit that is a flame of God abides,
A fiery portion of the Wonderful,
Artist of his own beauty and delight,
Immortal in our mortal poverty.

That is the consciousness of the jiva [soul], the personal, individual consciousness.

It is the individual consciousness. Aspiration is almost always an expression of the psychic being - the part of us that's organized around the divine center, the small divine flame deep within human beings. You see, this divine flame exists inside each human being, and little by little, through all the incarnations and karma and so on, a being takes shape around it, called the "psychic being." And when the psychic being reaches its full development, it becomes a kind of bodily or at any rate individual raiment of the soul. The soul is a portion of the Supreme - the jiva is the Supreme in individual form. And since there is only one Supreme, there is only one jiva, but with millions of individual forms. This jiva begins as a divine spark - immutable, eternal and infinite too (infinite in possibility rather than dimension). And through all the incarnations, whatever has received and responded to the divine Influence progressively crystallizes around the jiva, which becomes more and more conscious as well as more and more organized. Ultimately it becomes a completely conscious individual being, master of itself and moved exclusively by the divine Will. That is to say, an individual expression of the Supreme. This is what we call the «psychic being.»

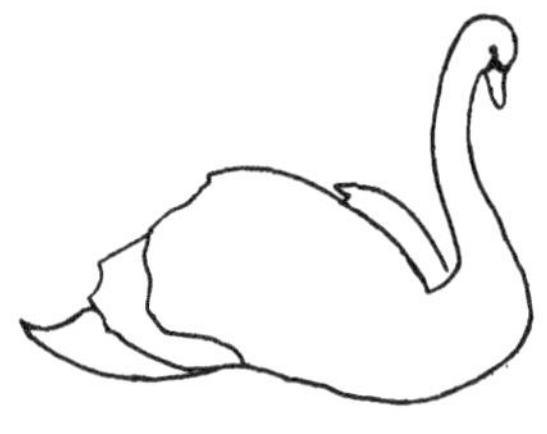

Power? It is usually the psychic which guides the being. One knows nothing about it because one is not conscious of it but usually it is that which guides the being. If one is very attentive, one becomes aware of it. But the majority of men haven't the least idea of it. For instance, when they have decided, in their outer ignorance, to do something, and instead of their being able to do it, all the circumstances are so organised that they do something else, they start shouting, storming, flying into a rage against fate, saying (that depends on what they believe, their beliefs) that Nature is wicked or their destiny baleful or God unjust, or... no matter what (it depends on what they believe). Whilst most of the time it is just the very circumstance which was most favourable for their inner development. And naturally, if you ask the psychic to help you to fashion a pleasant life for yourself, to earn money, have children who will be the pride of the family, etc., well, the psychic will not help you. But it will create for you all the circumstances necessary to awaken something in you so that the need of union with the Divine may be born in your consciousness. At times you have made fine plans, and if they had succeeded, you would have been more and more encrusted in your outer ignorance, your stupid little ambition and your aimless activity. Whilst if you receive a good shock, and the post you coveted is denied to you, the plan you made is shattered, and you find yourself completely thwarted, then, sometimes this opposition opens to you a door on something truer and deeper. And when you are a little awake and look back, if you are in the least sincere, you say: "Ah! It wasn't I who was right — it was Nature or the divine Grace or my psychic being who did it." It is the psychic being which organised that.

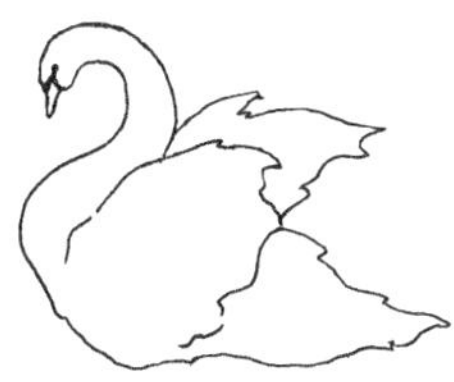

Man's hopes and longings build the journeying wheels
That bear the body of his destiny
And lead his blind will towards an unknown goal.
His fate within him shapes his acts and rules;
Its face and form already are born in him,
Its parentage is in his secret soul:
Here Matter seems to mould the body's life
And the soul follows where its nature drives.
Nature and Fate compel his free-will's choice.
But greater spirits this balance can reverse
And make the soul the artist of its fate.
This is the mystic truth our ignorance hides:
Doom is a passage for our inborn force,
Our ordeal is the hidden spirit's choice,
Ananke is our being's own decree.

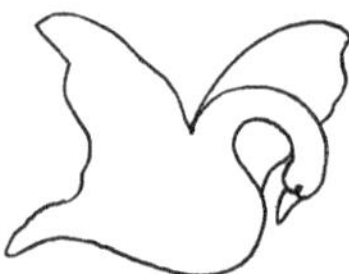

*Mother, here Sri Aurobindo speaks of "the psychic behind
supporting all". What does this mean?*

Well, yes, the psychic is behind the whole organisation, this
triple organisation of human life and consciousness, the
psychic is behind and supports it by its consciousness which
is an immortal one. It is because of the psychic that we have
so clear a sense of continuity. Otherwise if you compare what
you now are with what you were when you were three,
obviously you couldn't recognise yourself in any way, either
physically or vitally or mentally. There is no resemblance of
any kind. But behind there is the psychic which supports the
development, the growth of the being and gives this continuity
of consciousness, makes one feel that he is the same being even
while being absolutely different, absolutely different. If later
one observes himself sufficiently, he can see that the things he
understood and could do at that time are things which seem to

him absolutely inconceivable now, and that he could never do a similar thing because he is no longer that person at all. And yet, because within there was the psychic consciousness which is immortal, one has the feeling that it is always the same being which was there and continues to be there with more or less progressive and more or less conscious changes.

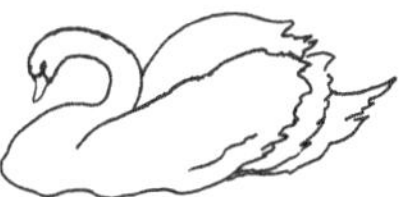

Our soul from its mysterious chamber acts;
Its influence pressing on our heart and mind
Pushes them to exceed their mortal selves.
It seeks for Good and Beauty and for God;
We see beyond self's walls our limitless self,
We gaze through our world's glass at half-seen vasts,
We hunt for the Truth behind apparent things.
Our inner Mind dwells in a larger light,
Its brightness looks at us through hidden doors;
Our members luminous grow and Wisdom's face
Appears in the doorway of the mystic ward:
When she enters into our house of outward sense,
Then we look up and see, above, her sun.

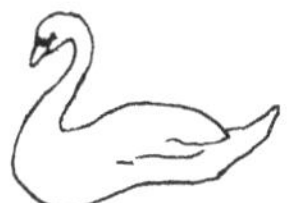

Does the psychic being identify itself with the inner truth?

It organises itself around it and enters into contact with it. The psychic is moved by the Truth. The Truth is something eternally self-existent and dependent on nothing in time or space, whereas the psychic being is a being that grows, takes form, progresses, individualises itself more and more. In this way it becomes more and more capable of manifesting this Truth, the eternal Truth that is one and permanent. The psychic being is a progressive being, which means that the relation between the psychic being and the Truth is a progressive one. It is not possible to become aware of one's psychic being without becoming aware at the same time of the inner Truth. All those who have had this experience — not a mental experience but an integral experience of contact with the psychic being, not a contact with the idea they have constructed of it, but a truly concrete contact — all say the same thing: from the very minute this contact takes place, one is absolutely conscious of the eternal Truth within oneself and one sees that it is the purpose of life and the guide of the world.

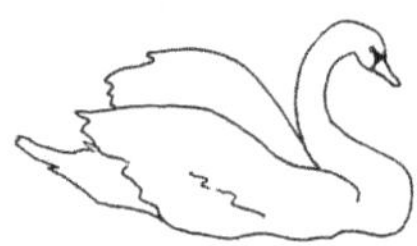

To want what the Divine wants in all sincerity is the essential condition for peace and joy in life. Almost all human miseries come from the fact that human beings are almost always persuaded they know better than the Divine what they need and what life is supposed to bring them. The majority of human beings want other human beings to behave according to their own expectations and life circumstances to follow their own desires, hence they suffer and are unhappy.

Only by giving oneself in all sincerity to the Divine Will does one gain the peace and calm joy that arises from the abolition of desires.

The psychic being knows this definitely. Thus, by uniting with our psychic being, we can know it, too. But the first condition is not to be the slave of personal desires and mistake them for the truth of one's being.

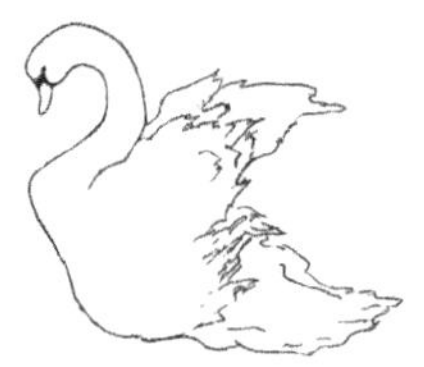

It is always pure. But it is more or less individualized and
independent in its action. What is psychic in the being is
always pure, by its very definition, for it is that part of the being
which is in contact with the Divine and expresses the truth of
the being. But this may be like a spark in the darkness of the
being, or it may be a being of light, conscious, fully formed and
independent. There are all the gradations between the two.

It is the outer consciousness that is not in contact with it, for it is
turned outwards instead of being turned inwards – for it lives
amidst all the external noise and movements, in what it sees,
what it does, what it says, instead of looking within, into the
depths of the being and listening to the inner inspiration.

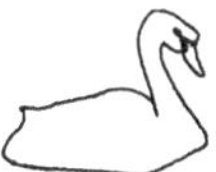

Unseen, a captive in a house of sound,
The spirit lost in the splendour of a dream
Listens to a thousand-voiced illusion's ode.
A delicate weft of sorcery steals the heart
Or a fiery magic tints her tones and hues,
Yet they but wake a thrill of transient grace;
A vagrant march struck by the wanderer Time,
They call to a brief unsatisfied delight
Or wallow in ravishments of mind and sense,
But miss the luminous answer of the soul.

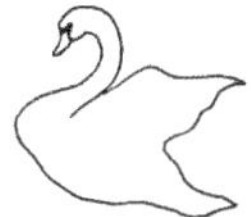

The soul, the psychic being is in direct touch with the divine
Truth, but it is hidden in man by the mind, the vital being and the
physical nature. One may practice yoga and get illuminations in
the mind and the reason; one may conquer power and luxuriate

in all kinds of experiences in the vital: one may establish even surprising physical Siddhis; but if the true soul- power behind does not manifest, if the psychic nature does not come into the front, nothing genuine has been done. In this yoga the psychic being is that which opens the rest of the nature to the true supramental light and finally to the supreme Ananda. Mind can open by itself to its own higher reaches: it can still itself and widen into the Impersonal: it may too spiritualise itself in some kind of static liberation or Nirvana: but the supramental cannot find a sufficient base in a spiritualised mind alone. If the inmost soul is awakened, if there is a new birth out of the mere mental, vital and physical into the psychic consciousness, then this yoga can be done; otherwise (by the sole power of the mind or any other part) it is impossible.

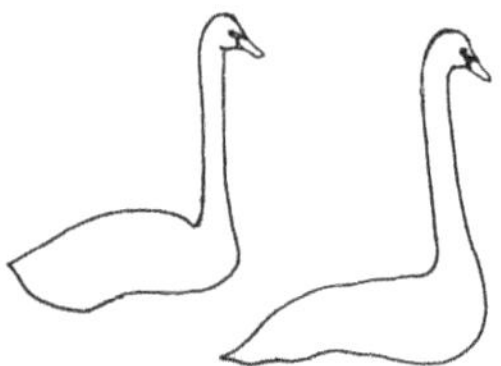

"Happy are they who in this chaos of things,
This coming and going of the feet of Time,
Can find the single Truth, the eternal Law:
Untouched they live by hope and doubt and fear.
Happy are men anchored on fixed belief
In this uncertain and ambiguous world,
Or who have planted in the heart's rich soil
One small grain of spiritual certitude.
Happiest who stand on faith as on a rock.
But I must pass leaving the ended search,
Truth's outcome firm, unmutable
And this harmonic building of world-fact,
This ordered knowledge of apparant things.
Here I can stay not, for I seek my soul."

I think the more psychic one is, usually, the more difficulties he has. Only, one is armed to face the difficulties. But the more psychic one is, the more is he in contradiction with the present state of the world. So when one is in opposition with something, the result is difficulties. And I have noticed that most often those who have many difficulties are those who are in a more or less close contact with their psychic being. If you want to speak about outer circumstances — I am not speaking of the character, that's quite different, but of outer circumstances — the people who have to struggle most and would have most reason to suffer are those who have a very developed psychic being.

First, the development of the psychic being has a double result which is concomitant. That is, with the development of the psychic being, the sensitivity of the being grows. And with the growth of sensitivity there is also the growth of the capacity for suffering; but there is the counterpart, that is, to the extent to which one is in relation with the psychic being, one faces the circumstances of life in an altogether different way and with a kind of inner freedom which makes one capable of withdrawing from a circumstance and not feeling the shock in the ordinary way. You can face the difficulty or outer things with calm, peace, and a sufficient inner knowledge not to be troubled. So, on one side you are more sensitive and on the other you have more strength to deal with the sensitivity.

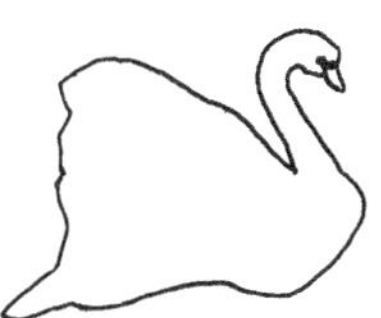

Generally speaking, those who practice yoga have either a fully developed, independent psychic being which has taken birth again to do the Divine's work, or else a psychic being in its last incarnation wanting to complete its development and realize itself.

This is what aspires, this is what has the contact.

So, when you're told "become conscious of your psychic being," it's for the being formed by external Nature to contact the divine Presence through the psychic being. Then the psychic takes charge of the whole being; in fact, it is the inner Guide.... Well, when I was a little child, this "person" (which wasn't a person, but an expression of a certain consciousness and will) was actually the psychic presence; there was something else behind, but that's a rather special case. And what happened to me happens to everyone whose psychic being has deliberately incarnated: the psychic being guides your life, and if you let it act freely, it arranges ALL circumstances - it's truly wonderful! ... I have seen - not only for myself but for so many people who also had conscious psychic beings - that everything is arranged with a view to ... not at all your personal egoistic satisfaction, but your ultimate progress and realization. And all circumstances of life, even those you call "disastrous," are there to lead you where you have to go as swiftly as possible.

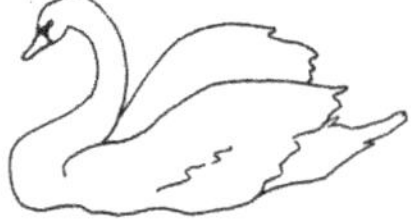

When someone is destined for the Path, all circumstances through all the deviations of mind and life help in one way or another to lead him to it. It is his own psychic being within him and Divine Power above that use to that end the vicissitudes both of mind and outward circumstance.

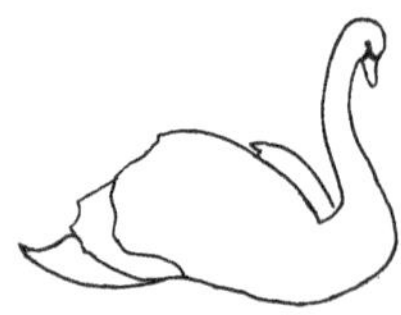

Each of you should be able to get into touch with your own psychic being, it is not an inaccessible thing. Your psychic being is there precisely to put you in contact with the divine forces. And if you are in contact with your psychic being, you begin to

feel, to have a kind of perception of what divine love can be…
It is not enough that one morning you wake up saying "Oh! I would like to be in contact with divine Love", it is not like that. If, through a sustained effort, a deep concentration, a great forgetfulness of self, you succeed in coming into touch with your psychic being, you will never dream of thinking, "Oh! I would like to be in contact with divine Love" — you are in a state in which everything appears to you to be this divine Love and nothing else. And yet it is only a covering, but a covering of a beautiful texture.

So, divine Love need not be sought and known apart from the psychic being?

No. find your psychic being and you will understand what divine Love is. Do not try to come into direct contact with divine Love because this will yet again be a vital desire pushing you: you will perhaps not be aware of it, but it will be a vital desire.

You must make an effort to come into touch with your psychic being, to become aware and free in the consciousness of your psychic being, and then, quite naturally, spontaneously, you will know what divine Love is.

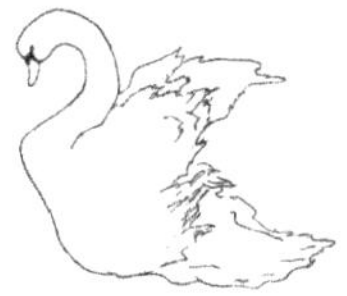

The source of sincerity, of will, of perseverance is in the psychic being, but this translates itself differently in different people.

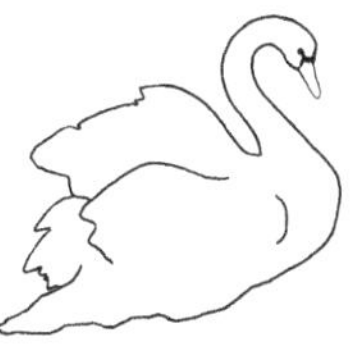

The complete unification of the whole being around the psychic centre is the essential condition to realize a perfect sincerity.

"Remember why thou cam'st:
Find out thy soul, recover thy hid self,
In silence seek God's meaning in thy depths,
Then mortal nature change to the divine.
Open God's door, enter into his trance..."   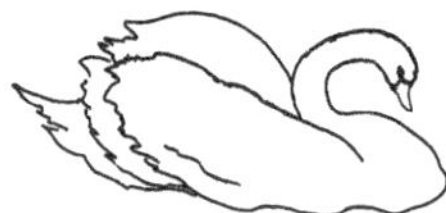

Purification and consecration are two great necessities of sadhana. Those who have experiences before purification run a great risk: it is much better to have the heart pure first, for then the way becomes safe. That is why I advocate the psychic change of the nature first — for that means the purification of the heart: the turning of it wholly to the Divine, the subjection of the mind and the vital to the control of the inner being, the soul. Always, when the soul is in front, one gets the right guidance from within as to what is to be done, what avoided, what is the wrong thing or the true thing in thought, feeling, action. But this inner intimation emerges in proportion as the consciousness grows more and more pure.

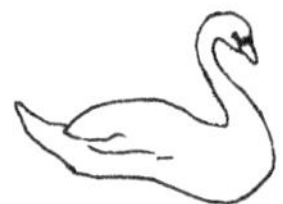

The soul is always pure, but the knowledge and force in it are involved and come out only as the psychic being evolves and grows stronger.

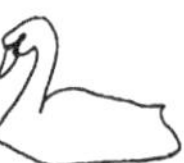

What characterizes the substance of the psychic world?

The substance of the psychic world is a substance proper to it, with its own psychic characteristics: a sense of immortality, a complete receptivity to the divine influence, an entire submission to this influence by which it is wholly impregnated. It is this exactly which distinguishes the psychic from the other parts of the being. When, for instance, I speak of organising the mind and the vital around the psychic centre, I do not mean that they become psychic; they remain the mind and the vital, but they are organised around the psychic as an army is organised around its leader — it does not become the leader, it obeys him, doesn't it? Well, it is the same thing here; the vital and the mind are organised around the psychic, they receive orders from the psychic and carry them out as well as they can. But their substance does not become psychic substance as a consequence. They can be under the intluence of the psychic and assume its nature more or less but not its substance.

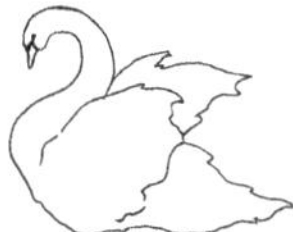

Indeed, the expression of a true psychic life in the being is peace, a joyful serenity. Any suffering is therefore a precious indication to us of our weak point, of the point which demands a greater spiritual effort from us.

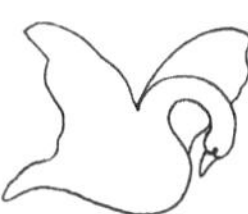

Sweet Mother, can the psychic express itself without the mind, the vital and the physical?

It expresses itself constantly without them. Only, in order that the ordinary human being may perceive it, it has to express itself through them, because the ordinary human being is not in direct contact with the psychic. If it was in direct contact with the psychic it would be psychic in its manifestation — and all would be truly well. But as it is not in contact with the psychic it doesn't even know what it is, it wonders all bewildered what kind of a being it can be; so to reach this ordinary human consciousness it must use ordinary means, that is, go through the mind, the vital and the physical.

One of them may be skipped but surely not the last, otherwise one is no longer conscious of anything at all.

It is the action of the psychic being, not the being itself, that gets mixed with the mental, vital and physical disabilities because it has to use them to express what little of the true psychic feeling gets through the veil. It is by the heart's aspiration to the Divine that the psychic being gets free from these disabilities.

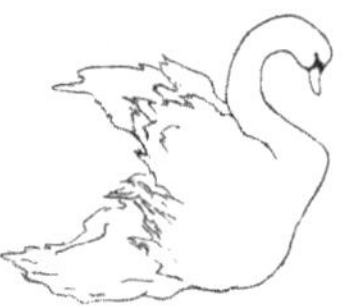

These things, anger, jealousy, desire are the very stuff of the ordinary human vital consciousness. They could not be changed if there were not a deeper consciousness within which is of quite another character. There is within you a psychic being which is divine, directly a part of the Mother, pure of all these defects. It is covered and concealed by the ordinary consciousness and nature, but when it is unveiled and able to come forward and govern the being, then it changes the ordinary consciousness, throws all these undivine things out and changes the outer nature altogether. That is why we want the sadhaks to concentrate, to open this concealed consciousness — it is by concentration of whatever kind and the experiences it brings that one opens and becomes aware within and the new consciousness and nature begin to grow and come out. Of course we want them also to use their will and reject the desires and wrong movements of the vital, for by doing that the emergence of the true consciousness becomes possible. But rejection alone cannot succeed: it is by rejection and by inner experience and growth that it is done.

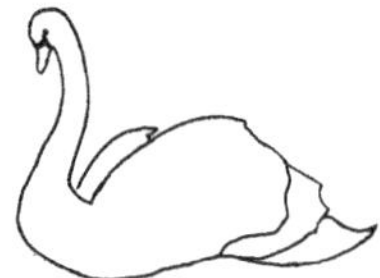

Compassion and gratitude are essentially psychic virtues. They appear in the consciousness only when the psychic being takes part in active life.

Sweet Mother, Does an outer life of evil deeds and a base consciousness have an effect on the psychic being? Is there a possibility of its degradation?

A base and evil life can only have the effect of separating the outer being more and more completely from the psychic being, which retires into the depths of the higher consciousness and sometimes even cuts off all relation with the body, which is then usually possessed by an asuric or rakshasic being.

The psychic being itself is above all possibility of degradation.

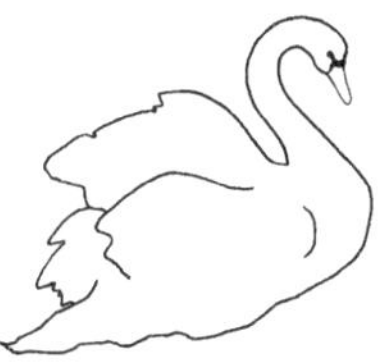

A TREE

A tree beside the sandy river-beach
    Holds up its topmost boughs
Like fingers towards the skies they cannot reach,
    Earth-bound, heaven-amorous.

This is the soul of man. Body and brain
Hungry for earth our heavenly flight detain. 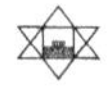

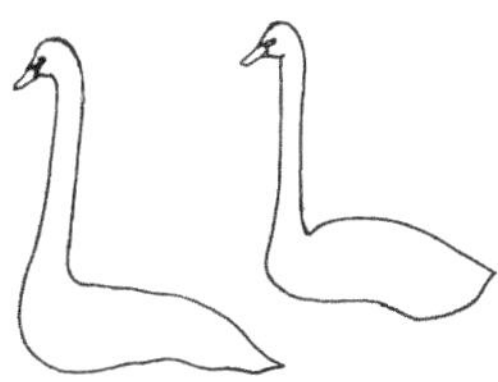

The inferior nature born into ignorance
Still took too large a place, it veiled her self
And must be pushed aside to find her soul. 

All that comes from the mind is wholly relative. The more the mind is educated and has applied itself to various disciplines, the more it becomes capable of proving that what it puts forward or what it says is true. One can prove the truth of anything by reasoning, but that does not make it true. It remains an opinion, a prejudice, a knowledge based on appearances which are themselves more than dubious.

So there seems to be only one way out and that is to go in search of one's soul and to find it. It is there, it does not make a point of hiding itself it does not play with you just to make things difficult; on the contrary, it makes great efforts to help you find it and to make itself heard. Only between your soul and your active consciousness there are two characters who are in the habit of making a lot of noise, the mind and the vital. And because they make a lot of noise, while the soul does not, or, rather, makes as little as possible, their noise prevents you from hearing the voice of the soul.

When you want to know what your soul knows, you have to make an inner effort, to be very attentive: and indeed, if you are attentive, behind the outer noise of the mind and the vital, you can discern something very subtle, very quiet, very peaceful, which knows and says what it knows. But the insistence of the others is so imperious, while that is so quiet, that you are very easily misled into listening to the one that makes the most noise; most often you become aware only afterwards that the other one was right. It does not impose itself, it does not compel you to listen, for it is without violence.

When you hesitate, when you wonder what to do in this or that circumstance, there comes the desire, the preference both mental and vital, that press, insist, affirm and impose themselves, and, with the best reasons in the world, build up a whole case for themselves. And if you are not on the alert, if you don't have a firm discipline, if you don't have the habit of control, they finally convince you that they are right. And they make so much noise that you do not even hear the tiny voice or the tiny, very quiet indication of the soul which says, "Don't do it."

This "Don't do it" comes often, but you discard it as something which has no power and follow your impulsive destiny. But if you are truly sincere in your will to find and live the truth, then you learn to listen better and better, you learn to discriminate more and more, and even if it costs you an effort, even if it causes you pain, you learn to obey. And even if you have obeyed only once, it is a powerful help, a considerable progress on the path towards the discrimination between what is and what is not the soul. With this discrimination and the necessary sincerity you are sure to reach the goal.

But you must not be in a hurry, you must not be impatient, you must be very persevering. You do the wrong thing ten times for every time that you do the right thing. But when you do the wrong thing you must not give up everything in despair, but tell yourself that the Grace will never abandon you and that next time it will be better.

So, in conclusion, we shall say that in order to know things as they are you must first unite with your soul and to unite with your soul you must want it with persistence and perseverance.

Only the degree of concentration on the goal can shorten the way.

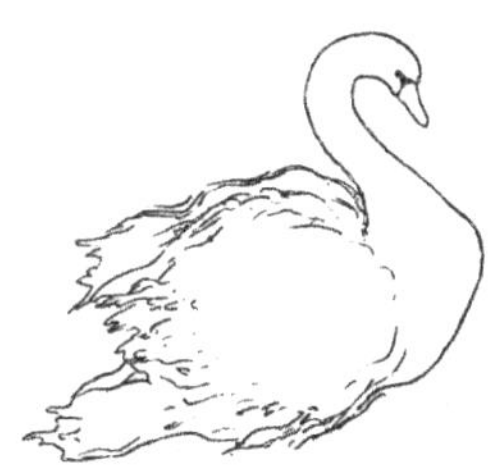

But now her spirit's flame of conscient force
Retiring from a sweetness without fruit
Called back her thoughts from speech to sit within
In a deep room in meditation's house.
For only there could dwell the soul's firm truth:
Imperishable, a tongue of sacrifice,
It flamed unquenched upon the household hearth
Where burns for the high houselord and his mate
The homestead's sentinel and witness fire
From which the altars of the gods are lit.

SURRENDER

O Thou of whom I am the instrument,
        O secret Spirit and Nature housed in me,
Let all my mortal being now be blent
        In thy still glory of divinity.

I have given my mind to be dug Thy channel mind,
        I have offered up my will to be Thy will:
Let nothing of myself be left behind
        In our union mystic and unutterable.

My heart shall throb with the world-beats of Thy love,
        My body become Thy engine for earth-use:
In my nerves and veins Thy rapture's streams shall move;
    My thoughts shall be hounds of Light for Thy power to loose.

    Keep only my soul to adore eternally
    And meet Thee in each form and soul of Thee.   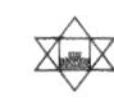

It is not the psychic being that suffers for personal reasons, it is
the mind, the vital and the ordinary consciousness of ignorant
man. This is because the contact between the outer consciousness
and the psychic consciousness is not well established. He in
whom the contact has been well established is always happy.

The psychic being works with perseverance and ardour
for the union to be made an accomplished fact, but it never
complains and knows how to wait for the hour of realisation
to come.

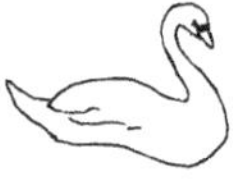

True happiness does not depend on the external circumstances
of life. One can obtain true happiness and keep it constantly
only by discovering one's psychic being and uniting with it.

The realisation of the psychic being, its awakening and the bringing of it in front depend mainly on the extent to which one can develop a personal relation with the Divine, a relation of Bhakti, love, reliance, self-giving, rejection of the insistences of the separating and self-asserting mental, vital and physical ego. 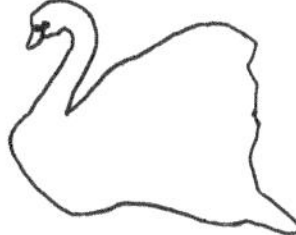

A mystic slow transfiguration works.
All our earth starts from mud and ends in sky,
And Love that was once an animal's desire,
Then a sweet madness in the rapturous heart,
An ardent comradeship in the happy mind,
Becomes a wide spiritual yearning's space.
A lonely soul passions for the Alone,
The heart that loved man thrills to the love of God, 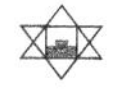

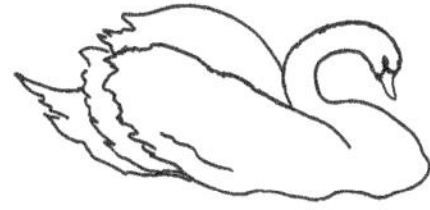

Sweet Mother,
Sri Aurobindo says that the voice of the ordinary conscience
is not the voice of the soul. What is it then?

The voice of the ordinary conscience is an ethical voice, a moral voice which distinguishes between good and evil, encourages us to do good and forbids us to do evil. This voice is very useful in ordinary life, until one is able to become conscious of one's psychic being and allow oneself to be entirely guided by it — in other words, to rise above ordinary humanity, free oneself from all egoism and become a conscious instrument of the Divine Will. The soul itself, being a portion of the Divine, is above all moral and ethical notions; it bathes in the Divine Light and manifests it, but it can truly govern the whole being only when the ego has been dissolved.

The mental being within watches, observes and passes judgment on all that happens in you. The psychic does not watch and observe in this way like a witness, but it feels and knows spontaneously in a much more direct and luminous way, by the very purity of its own nature and the divine instinct within it, and so, whenever it comes to the front it reveals at once what are the right and what the wrong movements in your nature.

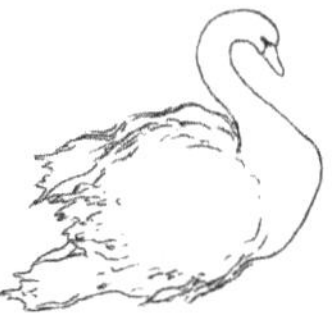

You say that it is necessary to establish "homogeneity in our being"?

Don't you know what a homogeneous thing is, made up of all similar parts? That means the whole being must be under the same influence, same consciousness, same tendency, same will. We are formed of all kinds of different pieces. They become active one after another. According to the part that is active, one is quite another person, becomes almost another personality. For instance, one had an aspiration at first, felt that everything existed only for the Divine, then something happens, somebody comes along, one has to do something, and everything disappears. One tries to recall the experience, not even the memory of the experience remains. One is completely under another influence, one wonders how this could have happened…I am speaking about something which has happened to all of you: you have had an experience, and for some time you have felt, understood that this experience was the only thing that was important, that had an absolute value — half an hour later you try to recall it, it is like a smoke that vanishes. The experience has disappeared. And yet half an hour ago it was there and so powerful.... It is because one is made of all kinds of different things. The body is like a bag with pebbles and pearls all mixed up, and it is only the bag which keeps all that together. This is not a homogeneous, uniform consciousness but a heterogeneous one.

You can be a different person at different moments in your life. I know people who took decisions, had a strong will, knew what they wanted and prepared to do it. Then there is a little reversal in the being; another part came up and spoilt all the work in ten minutes. What had been accomplished in two months was all undone. When the first part comes back it is in dismay, it says: "What!.. ." Then the whole work has to be started again, slowly. Hence it is evident that it is very important to become aware of the psychic being; one must have a kind of signpost or a mirror in which all things are reflected and show themselves as they truly are. And then, according to what they are, one puts them in one place or another; one begins to explain, to organise. That takes time. The same part comes back three or four times and every part that comes up says: "Put me in the first place; what the others do is not important, not at all important, it is I who will decide, for I am the most important." I am sure that if you look at yourself, you will see that there's not one among you who has not had the experience. You want to become conscious, to have goodwill, you have understood, your aspiration is shining — all is brilliant, illuminated; but all of a sudden something happens, a useless conversation, some unfortunate reading, and that upsets everything. Then one thinks that it was an illusion one lived in, that all things were seen from a certain angle.

This is life. One stumbles and falls at the first occasion. One tells oneself: "Oh! One can't always be so serious", and when the other part returns, once again, one repents bitterly: "I was a fool, I have wasted my time, now I must begin again...." At times there is one part that's ill-humoured, in revolt, full of worries, and another which is progressive, full of surrender. All that, one after the other.

There is but one remedy: that signpost must always be there, a mirror well placed in one's feelings, impulses, all one's sensations. One sees them in this mirror. There are some which are not very beautiful or pleasant to look at; there are others which are beautiful, pleasant, and must be kept. This one does a hundred times a day if necessary. And it is very interesting. One draws a kind of big circle around the psychic mirror and arranges all the elements around it. If there is something that is not all right, it casts a sort of grey shadow upon the mirror: this element must be shifted, organised. It must be spoken to, made to understand, one must come out of that darkness. If you do that, you never get bored. When people are not kind, when one has a cold in the head, when one doesn't know one's lessons, and so on, one begins to look into this mirror. It is very interesting, one sees the canker. "I thought I was sincere!" — not at all.

Not a thing happens in life which is not interesting. This mirror is very, very well made. Do that for two years, three, four years, at times one must do it for twenty years. Then at the end of a few years, look back, turn your gaze upon what you were three years ago: "How I have changed!... Was I like that?… But I was indeed stupid! How I have changed!" Isn't it very interesting, isn't it?

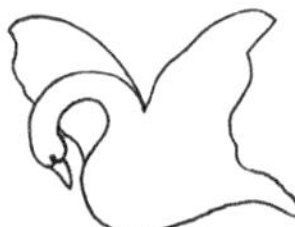

The work of unifying the being consists of:
(1) becoming aware of one's psychic being.
(2) Putting before the psychic being, as one becomes aware of them, all one's movements, impulses, thoughts and acts of will, so that the psychic being may accept or reject each of these movements, impulses, thoughts or acts of will. Those that are accepted will be kept and carried out; those that are rejected will be driven out of the consciousness so that they may never come back again.

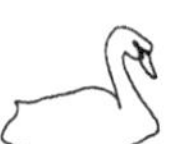

'The complete unification of the whole being around the psychic center is the essential condition to realize a perfect sincerity.'

I have noticed that people are insincere simply because one part of their being says one thing and another part says something else. That's what causes insincerity. It came very clearly: a vision, you know, an inner vision. So I tried to put it down on paper; I don't know if it's clear.

The psychic being is in the heart centre in the middle of the chest (not in the physical heart, for all the centres are in the middle of the body), but it is deep behind. When one is going away from the vital into the psychic, it is felt as if one is going deep deep down till one reaches that central place of the psychic. The surface of the heart centre is the place of the emotional being; from there one goes deep to find the psychic. 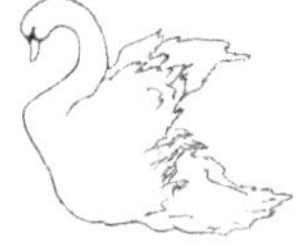

"In Matter's body find thy heaven-born soul."
Then Savitri surged out of her body's wall
And stood a little span outside herself
And looked into her subtle being's depths
And in its heart as in a lotus-bud
Divined her secret and mysterious soul. 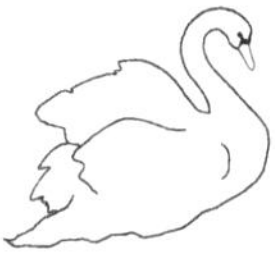

Is the psychic being in the heart?

Not in the physical heart, not in the organ. It is in a fourth dimension. an inner dimension. But it is in that region, the region somewhat behind the solar plexus, it is there that one finds it most easily. The psychic being is in the fourth dimension as related to our physical being. 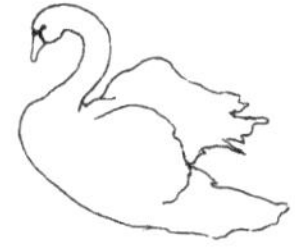

You have asked what is the discipline to be followed in order to convert the mental seeking into a living spiritual experience. The first necessity is the practice of concentration of your consciousness within yourself. The ordinary human mind has an activity on the surface which veils the real Self. But there is another, a hidden consciousness within behind the surface one in which we can become aware of the real Self and of a larger deeper truth of nature, can realise the Self and liberate and transform the nature. To quiet the surface mind and begin to live within is the object of this concentration. Of this true consciousness other than the superficial there are two main centres, one in the heart (not the physical heart, but the cardiac centre in the middle of the chest), one in the head.

The concentration in the heart opens within and by following this inward opening and going deep one becomes aware of the soul or psychic being, the divine element in the individual. This being unveiled begins to come forward, to govern the nature, to turn it and all its movements towards the Truth, towards the Divine, and to call down into it all that is above. It brings the consciousness of the Presence, the dedication of the being to the Highest and invites the descent into our nature of a greater Force and Consciousness which is waiting above us. To concentrate in the heart centre with the offering of oneself to the Divine and the aspiration for this inward opening and for the Presence in the heart is the first way and, if it can be done, the natural beginning; for its result once obtained makes the spiritual path far more easy and safe than if one begins the other way.

That other way is the concentration in the head, in the mental centre. This, if it brings about the silence of the surface mind, opens up an inner, larger, deeper mind within which is more capable of receiving spiritual experience and spiritual knowledge. But once concentrated here one must open the silent mental consciousness upward to all that is above mind. After a time one feels the consciousness rising upward and in the end it rises beyond the lid which has so long kept it tied in the body and finds a centre above the head where it is liberated into the Infinite. There it begins to come into contact with the universal Self, the Divine Peace, Light, Power, Knowledge, Bliss, to enter into that and become that, to feel the descent of these things into the nature. To concentrate in the head with the aspiration for quietude in the mind and the realisation of the Self and Divine above is the second way of concentration.

It is important, however, to remember that the concentration of the consciousness in the head is only a preparation for its rising to the centre above; otherwise, one may get shut up in one's own mind and its experiences or at best attain only to a reflection of the Truth above instead of rising into the spiritual transcendence to live there. For some the mental concentration is easier, for some the concentration in the heart centre; some are capable of doing both alternately — but to begin with the heart centre, if one can do it, is the more desirable.

The other side of discipline is with regard to the activities of the nature, of the mind, of the life-self or vital, of the physical being. Here the principle is to accord the nature with the inner realisation so that one may not be divided into two discordant parts. There are here several disciplines or processes possible. One is to offer all the activities to the Divine and call for the inner guidance and the taking up of one's nature by a Higher Power.

If there is the inward soul-opening, if the psychic being comes forward, then there is no great difficulty — there comes with it a psychic discrimination, a constant intimation, finally a governance which discloses and quietly and patiently removes all imperfections, brings the right mental and vital movements and reshapes the physical consciousness also.

Another method is to stand back detached from the movements of the mind, life, physical being, to regard their activities as only a habitual formation of general Nature in the individual imposed on us by past workings, not as any part of our real being; in proportion as one succeeds in this, becomes detached, sees mind and its activities as not oneself, life and its activities as not oneself, the body and its activities as not oneself, one becomes aware of an inner Being within us — inner mental, inner vital, inner physical — silent, calm, unbound, unattached, which reflects the true Self above and can be its direct representative; from this inner silent Being proceeds a rejection of all that is to be rejected, an acceptance only of what can be kept and transformed, an inmost Will to perfection or a call to the Divine Power to do at each step what is necessary for the change of the Nature. It can also open mind, life and body to the inmost psychic entity and its guiding influence or its direct guidance. In most cases these two methods emerge and work together and finally fuse into one. But one can begin with either the one that one feels most natural and easy to follow.

Finally, in all difficulties where personal effort is hampered, the help of the Teacher can intervene and bring about what is needed for the realisation or for the immediate step that is necessary.

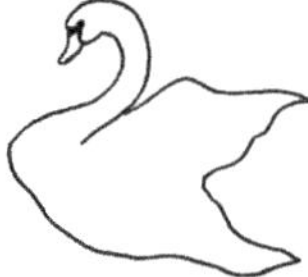

LILA

In us is the thousandfold Spirit who is one,
    An eternal thinker calm and great and wise,
A seer whose eye is an all-regarding sun,
    A poet of the cosmic mysteries.

A critic Witness pieces everything
    And binds the fragments in his brilliant sheaf:
A World-adventurer borne on Destiny's wing
    Gambles with death and triumph, joy and grief.

A king of greatness and a slave of love,
    Host of the stars and guest in Nature's inn,
A high spectator spirit throned above,
    A pawn of passion in the game divine.

One who has made in sport the suns and seas
Mirrors in our being his immense caprice.

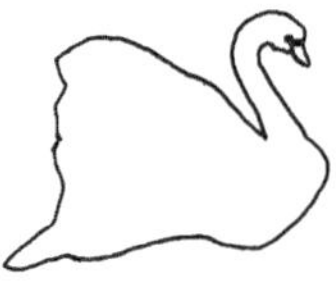

Aspiration, constant and sincere, and will to turn to the Divine alone are the best means to bring forward the psychic.

One can concentrate in any of the three centres which is easiest to the sadhak or gives most result. The power of the concentration in the heart-centre is to open that centre and by the power of aspiration, love, bhakti, surrender, remove the veil which covers and conceals the soul and bring forward the soul or psychic being to govern the mind, life and body and turn and open them all fully to the Divine, removing all that is opposed to that turning and opening.

This is what is called in this yoga the psychic transformation. The power of concentration above the head is to bring peace, silence, liberation from the body sense, the identification with mind and life and open the way for the lower (mental, vital, physical) consciousness to rise up to meet the higher consciousness above and for the powers of the higher (spiritual nature) consciousness to descend into mind, life and body. This is what is called in this yoga the spiritual transformation. If one begins with this movement then the Power from above has in its descent to open all the centres (including the lowest centre) and to bring out the psychic being; for until that is done there is likely to be much difficulty and struggle of the lower consciousness obstructing, mixing with or even refusing the Divine Action from above. If the psychic being is once active this struggle and these difficulties can be greatly minimised.

The power of concentration in the eyebrows is to open the centre there, liberate the inner mind and vision and the inner or yogic consciousness and its experiences and powers. From here also one can open upwards and act also in the lower centres; but the danger of this process is that one may get shut up in one's mental spiritual formations and not come out of them into the free and integral spiritual experience and knowledge and integral change of the being and nature.

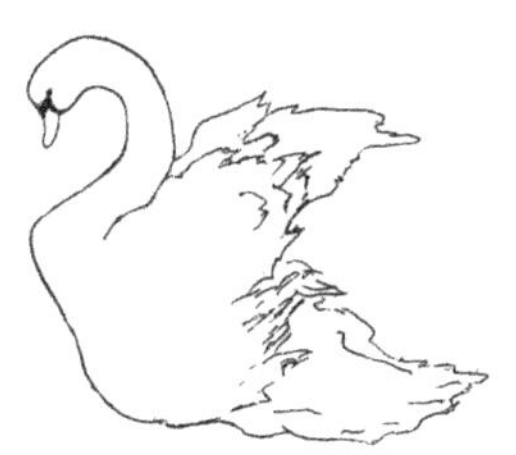

If the psychic is awake and in front, it becomes easy to remain conscious of the things that have to be changed in the external nature and it is comparatively easy to change them. But if the psychic gets veiled and retires in the background, the outer nature left to itself finds it difficult to remain conscious of its own wrong movements and even with great effort cannot succeed in getting rid of them. You can see yourself, as in the matter of the food, that with the psychic active and awake the right attitude comes naturally and whatever difficulty there was soon diminishes or even disappears.

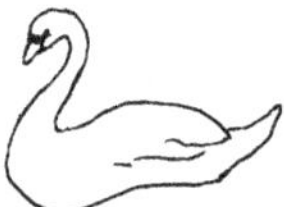

If desire is rejected and no longer governs the thought, feeling or action and there is a steady aspiration of an entirely sincere self-giving, the psychic usually after a time opens of itself.

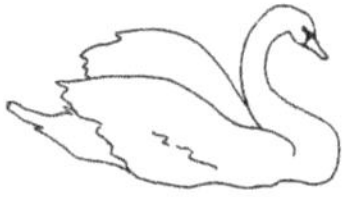

The emotional [devotion] is more outward than the psychic, it tends towards outward expression. The psychic is inwards and gives the direction to the whole inner and outer life. The emotional can be intense, but is neither so sure in its basis nor powerful enough to change the whole direction of the life.

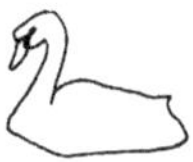

It is not the soul that suffers; the self is calm and equal to all things and the only sorrow of the psychic being is the sorrow of the resistance of Nature to the Divine Will or the resistance of things and people to the call of the True, the Good and the Beautiful. What is affected by suffering is the vital nature and the body. When the soul draws towards the Divine, there may be a resistance in the mind and the common form of that is denial and doubt — which may create mental and vital suffering. There may again be a resistance in the vital nature whose principal character is desire and the attachment to the objects of desire, and if in this field there is conflict between the soul and the vital nature, between the Divine Attraction and the pull of the Ignorance, then obviously there may be much suffering of the mind and vital parts. The physical consciousness also may offer a resistance which is usually that of a fundamental inertia, an obscurity in the very stuff of the physical, an incomprehension, an inability to respond to the higher consciousness, a habit of helplessly responding to the lower mechanically, even when it does not want to do so; both vital and physical suffering may be the consequence.

There is, moreover, the resistance of the Universal Nature which does not want the being to escape from the Ignorance into the Light. This may take the form of a vehement insistence in the continuation of the old movements, waves of them thrown on the mind and vital and body so that old ideas, impulses, desires, feelings, responses continue even after they are thrown out and rejected, and can return like an invading army from outside, until the whole nature, given to the Divine, refuses to admit them. This is the subjective form of the universal resistance, but it may also take an objective form, — opposition, calumny, attacks, persecution, misfortunes of many kinds, adverse conditions and circumstances, pain, illness, assaults from men or forces. There too the possibility of suffering is evident.

There are two ways to meet all that — first that of the Self, calm, equality, a spirit, a will, a mind, a vital, a physical consciousness that remain resolutely turned towards the Divine and unshaken by all suggestion of doubt, desire, attachment. depression, sorrow, pain, inertia.

This is possible when the inner being awakens, when one becomes conscious of the Self, of the inner Mind, the inner Vital, the inner Physical, for that can more easily attune itself to the divine Will, and then there is a division in the being as if there were two beings, one within, calm, strong. equal, unperturbed, a channel of the Divine Consciousness and Force, one without still encroached on by the lower Nature; but then the disturbances of the latter become something superficial which are no more than an outer ripple, — until these under the inner pressure fade and sink away and the outer being too remains calm, concentrated, unattackable.

There is also the way of the psychic, — when the psychic being comes out in its inherent power, its consecration, adoration, love of the divine, self- giving, surrender and imposes these on the mind, vital and physical consciousness and compels them to turn all their movements Godward. If the psychic is strong and master throughout, then there is no or little subjective suffering and the objective cannot affect either the soul or the other parts of the consciousness — the way is sunlit and a great joy and sweetness are the note of the whole sadhana.

As for the outer attacks and adverse circumstances, that depends on the action of the Force transforming the relations of the being with the outer Nature; as the victory of the Force proceeds, they will be eliminated; but however long they last, they cannot impede the sadhana, for then even adverse things and happenings become a means for its advance and for the growth of the spirit.

THE DUAL BEING

There are two beings in my single self.
    A Godhead watches Nature from behind
At play in front with a brilliant surface elf,
    A time-born creature with a human mind.

Tranquil and boundless like a sea or sky,
    The Godhead knows himself Eternity's son.
Radiant his mind and vast, his heart as free:
    His will is a sceptre of dominion.

The smaller self by Nature's passions driven,
    Thoughtful and erring learns his human task;
All must be known and to that greatness given
    His mind and life the mirror and the mask.

As with the figure of a symbol dance
The screened Omniscient plays at Ignorance.   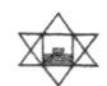

The psychic being emerges slowly in most men, even after taking up sadhana. There is so much in the mind and vital that has to change and readjust itself before the psychic can be entirely free. One has to wait till the necessary process has gone far enough before it can burst its agelong veil and come in front to control the nature. It is true that nothing can give so much inner happiness and joy — though peace can come by the mental and vital liberation or through the growth of a strong *samata* in the being.

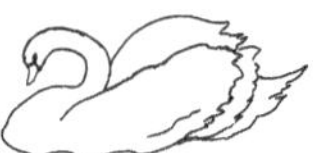

And I am sure that's how the work is done, slowly, imperceptibly, like a chick being formed in the egg: you see the shell, you see only the shell, you don't know what's inside, whether it's just an egg or a chick (normally, I mean - of course, you could see through with special instruments) and then the beak goes peck-peck! And then cheep! Out comes the chick, just like that. It's the same thing exactly for the contact with the psychic being. For months on end, sometimes years, you may be sitting before a closed door, push, push, pushing, and feeling, feeling the pressure (it hurts!), and there's nothing, no results. Then all at once, you don't know why or how, you sit down and poof! Everything bursts wide open, everything is ready, everything is done - it's over, you emerge into a full psychic consciousness and become intimate with your psychic being. Then everything changes - everything changes - your life completely changes, it's a total reversal of your whole existence.

In the end, it's best not to worry, not to get agitated or depressed (that's the worst of all), not to get worked up or impatient or disgusted - just be calm and say, "It will come when it comes," but with an unyielding stubbornness. Do what you feel has to be done, and keep on with it, keep on even if it seems utterly futile.

But if I only had a method!

There are methods - books are full of them. I don't recommend any of them: it's always the method the author uses or has heard of. Everyone has to find his own method. One can get certain hints, one can find one's own method.

The yoga is very usually a series of ups and downs till you get to a certain height. But there is a quite different reason for that — not the vagaries of the soul. On the contrary, when the psychic being gets in front and becomes master, there comes in a fundamentally smooth action and although there are difficulties and undulations of movement, these are no longer of an abrupt or dramatic character.

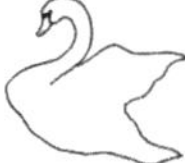

A secret soul behind supporting all
Is master and witness of our ignorant life,
Admits the Person's look and Nature's role.
But once the hidden doors are flung apart
Then the veiled king steps out in Nature's front;
A Light comes down into the Ignorance,
Its heavy painful knot loosens its grasp:
The mind becomes a mastered instrument
And life a hue and figure of the soul.
All happily grows towards knowledge and towards bliss.

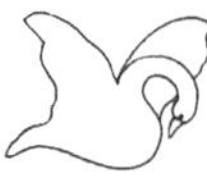

MOMENTS

If perfect moments on the peak of things,
    These tops of knowledge, greatness, ecstasy,
    Are only moments, this too enough might be.
I have put on the rapid flaming wings
Of souls whom the Ignorance black-robed Nature brings
    And the frail littleness of mortality
    Can bind not always. A high sovereignty
Makes them awhile creation's radiant kings.

These momentary upliftings of the soul
    Prepare the spirit's glorious permanence.
        The peace of God, a mighty transience,
Is now my spirit's boundless atmosphere.
    All parts are gathered into a timeless whole;
        All moments blaze in an eternal year. 

If you have within you a psychic being sufficiently awake to watch over you, to prepare your path, it can draw towards you things which help you, draw people, books, circumstances, all sorts of little coincidences which come to you as though brought by some benevolent will and give you an indication, a help, a support to take decisions and turn you in the right direction. But once you have taken this decision, once you have decided to find the truth of your being, once you start sincerely on the road, then everything seems to conspire to help you to advance.

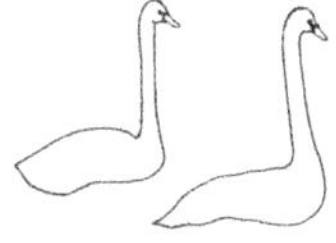

Is there a difference between the "spiritual" and the "psychic"? Are they different planes"?

Yes, the psychic plane belongs to the personal manifestation; the psychic is that which is divine in you put out to be dynamic in the play. But when we speak of the spiritual we are thinking of something that is concentrated in the Divine rather than in the external manifestation. The spiritual plane is something static behind and above the outward play; it supports the instruments of the nature, but is not itself included or involved in the external manifestation here.

But in speaking of these things one must be careful not to be imprisoned by the words we use. When I speak of the psychic or the spiritual, I mean things that are very deep and real behind the flat surface of the words and intimately connected even in their difference. Intellectual definitions and distinctions are too external and rigid to seize the true truth of things.

The turn of the psychic is different from that of the overhead planes. It has less of greatness, power, wideness, more of a smaller sweetness, delicate beauty; there is an intense beauty of emotion, a fine subtlety of true perception, an intimate language.

35

The expression "sweetness and light" can very well be applied to the psychic as the kernel of its nature. The spiritual plane, when it takes up these things, gives them a wider utterance, a greater splendour of light, a stronger sweetness, a breath of powerful audacity, strength and space.

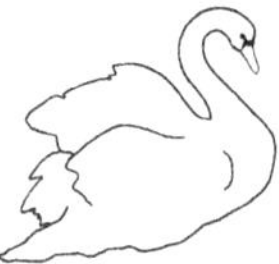

The silent Soul of all the world was there:
A Being lived, a Presence and a Power,
A single Person who was himself and all
And cherished Nature's sweet and dangerous throbs
Transfigured into beats divine and pure.
One who could love without return for love,
Meeting and turning to the best the worst,
It healed the bitter cruelties of earth,
Transforming all experience to delight;
Intervening in the sorrowful paths of birth
It rocked the cradle of the cosmic Child
And stilled all weeping with its hand of joy;
It led things evil towards their secret good,
It turned racked falsehood into happy truth;
Its power was to reveal divinity.

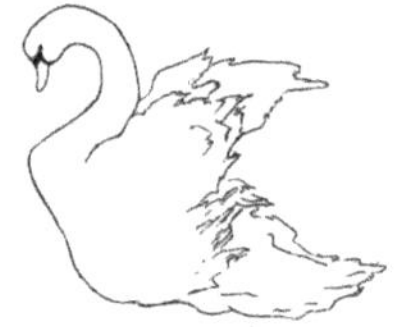

The psychic being stands behind mind, life and body, supporting them; so also the psychic world is not one world in the scale like the mental, vital or physical worlds, but stands behind all these and it is there that the souls evolving here retire for the time between life and life.

If the psychic were only one principle in the rising order of body, life and mind on a par with the others and placed somewhere in the scale on the same footing as the others, it could not be the soul of all the rest, the divine element making the evolution of the others possible and using them as instruments for a growth through cosmic experience towards the Divine. So also the psychic world cannot be one among the other worlds to which the evolutionary being goes for supraphysical experience; it is a plane where it retires into itself for rest, for a spiritual assimilation of what it has experienced and for a replunging into its own fundamental consciousness and psychic nature. 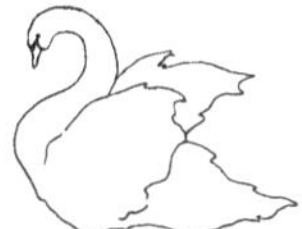

Immersed in voiceless internatal trance
The beings that once wore forms on earth sat there
In shining chambers of spiritual sleep.
Passed were the pillar-posts of birth and death,
Passed was their little scene of symbol deeds,
Passed were the heavens and hells of their long road;
They had returned into the world's deep soul.
All now was gathered into pregnant rest:
Person and nature suffered a slumber change.
In trance they gathered back their bygone selves,
In a background memory's foreseeing muse
Prophetic of new personality
Arranged the map of their coming destiny's course:
Heirs of their past, their future's discoverers,
Electors of their own self-chosen lot,
They waited for the adventure of new life. 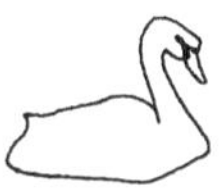

The Soul takes birth each time, and each time a mind, life and body are formed out of the materials of universal nature according to the soul's past evolution and its need for the future.

When the body is dissolved, the vital goes into the vital plane and remains there for a time, but after a time the vital sheath disappears. The last to dissolve is the mental sheath. Finally the soul or psychic being retires into the psychic world to rest there till a new birth is close.

This is the general course for ordinarily developed human beings. There are variations according to the nature of the individual and his development. For example, if the mental is strongly developed, then the mental being can remain; so also can the vital, provided they are organized by and centred around the true psychic being; they share the immortality of the psychic.

The soul gathers the essential elements of its experiences in life and makes that its basis of growth in the evolution; when it returns to birth it takes up with its mental, vital, physical sheaths so much of its Karma as is useful to it in the new life for further experience.

It is really for the vital part of the being that *sraddha* and rites are done — to help the being to get rid of the vital vibrations which still attach it to the earth or to the vital worlds, so that it may pass quickly to its rest in the psychic peace.

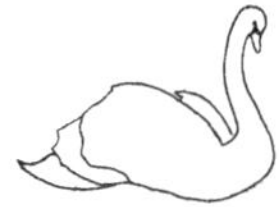

A Person persistent through the lapse of worlds,
Although the same for ever in many shapes
By the outward mind unrecognisable,
Assuming names unknown in unknown climes
Imprints through Time upon the earth's worn page
A growing figure of its secret self,
And learns by experience what the spirit knew,
Till it can see its truth alive and God.
Once more they must face the problem-game of birth,
The soul's experiment of joy and grief
And thought and impulse lighting the blind act,
And venture on the roads of circumstance,
Through inner movements and external scenes
Travelling to self across the forms of things.

There is another [remedy for fear of dying]. a little more difficult, but better, I believe. It lies in telling oneself: "This body is not I" and in trying to find in oneself the part which is truly one's self, until one has found one's psychic being. And when one has found one's psychic being — immediately, you understand — one has the sense of immortality. And one knows that what goes out or what comes in is just a matter of convenience: "I am not going to weep over a pair of shoes I put aside when it is full of holes! When my pair of shoes is worn out I cast it aside, and I do not weep." Well, the psychic being has taken this body because it needed to use it for its work, but when the time comes to leave the body, that is to say, when one must leave it because it is no longer of any use for some reason or other, one leaves the body and has no fear. It is quite a natural gesture — and it is done without the least regret, that's all.

And the moment you are in your psychic being, you have that feeling, spontaneously, effortlessly. You soar above the physical life and have the sense of immortality. As for me, I consider this the best remedy. The other is an intellectual, common-sense, rational remedy. This is a deep experience and you can always get it back as soon as you recover the contact with your psychic being. This is a truly interesting phenomenon, for it is automatic. The moment you are in contact with your psychic being, you have the feeling of immortality, of having always been and being always, eternally. And then what comes and goes – these are life's accidents, they have no importance.

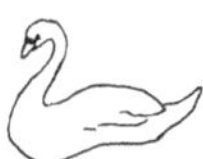

> In her beginningless infinity
> Through her soul's reaches unconfined she gazed;
> She saw the undying fountains of her life,
> She knew herself eternal without birth.

As the evolving being develops still more and becomes more rich and complex, it accumulates its personalities, as it were.

Sometimes they stand behind the active elements, throwing in some colour, some trait, some capacity here and there. — or they stand in front and there is a multiple personality, a many-sided character or a many-sided, sometimes what looks like a universal capacity. But if a former personality, a former capacity is brought fully forward, it will not be to repeat what was already done, but to cast the same capacity into new forms and new shapes and fuse it into a new harmony of the being which will not be a reproduction of what was before. Thus you must not expect to be what the warrior and the poet were. Something of the outer characteristics may reappear but very much changed and new-cast in a new combination. It is in a new direction that the energies will be guided to do what was not done before.

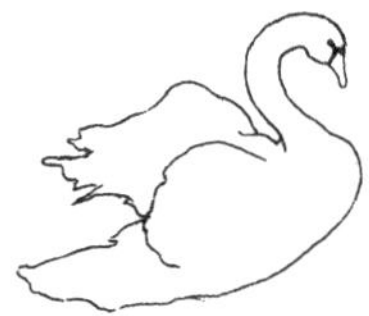

Into creation's centre he had come.
The spirit wandering from state to state
Finds here the silence of its starting-point
In the formless force and the still fixity
And brooding passion of the world of Soul.
All that is made and once again unmade,
The calm persistent vision of the One
Inevitably re-makes, it lives anew:
Forces and lives and beings and ideas
Are taken into the stillness for a while;
There they remould their purpose and their drift,
Recast their nature and re-form their shape.
Ever they change and changing ever grow,
And passing through a fruitful stage of death
And after long reconstituting sleep
Resume their place in the process of the Gods
Until their work in cosmic Time is done.

Only when one is consciously identified with one's divine origin, can one in truth speak of a memory of past lives. Sri Aurobindo speaks of the progressive manifestation of the Spirit in the forms in which it dwells. When one reaches the summit of this manifestation, one has a vision that plunges down upon the way traversed and one remembers.

But this memory is not a thing of the mental kind. Those who claim to have been such a baron of the Middle Ages or such a person who lived at such a place and such a time, are fanciful, they are simply victims of their own mental imagination. In fact, what remains of past lives are not beautiful pictures in which you appear as a mighty lord in a castle or a victorious general at the head of an army — that is only romance. What remains is the memory of those instants when the psychic being emerged from the depths of your being and revealed itself to you — that is to say, the memory of those instants when you were wholly conscious. That growth of consciousness is progressively effectuated in the course of evolution, and the memory of past lives is generally limited to the critical moments of evolution, to the decisive turns that marked the progress of your consciousness.

At the time when you live such moments of your life, you do not care at all about remembering that you were Mr. X. such a person, living at such a place and in such an epoch; it is not the memory of your civic status that remains. On the contrary, you lose all consciousness of these petty external things, accessories and perishables, so that you may be wholly in the flare of the soul revelation or of the divine contact. When you remember such instants of your past lives, the memory is so intense that it seems to be still very close, still living, and much more living than most of the ordinary memories of our present life. At times, in dreams, when you come into contact with certain planes of consciousness, you may have memories of such intensity, such vibrant colour, so to say, even more intense than the colours and things of the physical world. For these are the moments of true consciousness, and everything then puts on an extraordinary brilliance, everything is vibrant, everything is imbued with a quality that escapes the ordinary eye.

These minutes of contact with the soul are often those that

mark a decisive turn of our life, a forward step, a progress in consciousness, and that frequently corresponds with a crisis, an extremely intense situation when there comes a call in the whole being, a call so strong that the inner consciousness pierces the layers of unconsciousness covering it and is revealed all luminous on the surface. This call of the being, when very strong, can also bring about the descent of a divine emanation, an individuality, a divine aspect which joins with your individuality at a given moment in order to do a given work, win a battle, express one thing or another. The work done, the emanation very often withdraws. Then one may retain the memory of the circumstances that were around those minutes of revelation or inspiration: one sees again the scenery, the colour of the dress that one had put on, the colour of one's own skin, the things about you at that time — all that is fixed indelibly with an extraordinary intensity, because the things of the ordinary life revealed themselves then in their true intensity and their true colour. The consciousness that reveals itself in you, reveals at the same time the consciousness that is in things. At times, with the help of these details you may reconstitute the age in which you lived or the action that you did, find out the country where you were; but it is very easy also to make a romance and take imagination for reality.

Yet you must not believe that all memories of past lives are those of moments of great crisis, of important mission or of revelation. Sometimes they are moments very simple, transparent, when an integral, a perfect harmony of the being was expressed. And that may correspond to altogether insignificant external situations.

Apart from the things that were in your immediate surrounding at that moment, apart from that moment of contact with your psychic being, nothing remains. Once the privileged moment passes, the psychic being plunges into an inner somnolence and the whole outer life melts into a grey monotony which does not leave any trace. Besides, it is almost the same phenomenon as what happens in the course of the life that you lead at present: apart from those exceptional moments when you are at the summit of your being, mental or vital or even physical, the rest of your life seems to melt in to a kind of neutral colour which has no great interest, when it matters little whether you were at such a place instead of being at another, whether you did this thing or that. If you try to look at your life all at once, in order to gather, as it were, its essence, the twenty or thirty or forty years behind you, you will see rise up spontaneously two or three images which were the true moments of your life; the rest is effaced. A kind of spontaneous choice works in your consciousness and there is a tremendous elimination. This will give you a little idea of what happens in regard to past lives: the choice of a few select moments and an immense elimination.

It is very true that the earliest lives are very rudimentary; very few things subsist out of that, scattered memories few and far between. But the more one progresses in consciousness, the more the psychic being is consciously associated with the outer activities; the memories grow in number and become more coherent and precise. But still, here also, the memory that remains is that of the contact with the soul and at times that of things which were associated with the psychic revelation — not the civic status or the changing scenes around. And this will explain to you why the so-called memories of past animal lives are the most fantastic: the divine spark in them is buried much too deep down to be able to come up consciously to the surface and be associated with the outer life. One must become a wholly conscious being, conscious in all its parts, totally united with one's divine origin before one can truly say that one remembers his past lives.

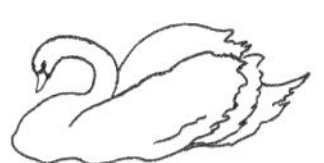

In rebirth it is not the external being, that which is formed by parents, environment and circumstances — the mental, the vital and the physical — that is born again: it is only the psychic being that passes from body to body. Logically then, neither the mental nor the vital being can remember past lives or recognise itself in the character or mode of life of this or that person. The psychic being alone can remember; and it is by becoming conscious of our psychic being that we can have at the same time exact impressions about our past lives.

That's not a psychic memory...it's when the vital, through some special circumstance, goes from one body to another, then it still remembers. That's generally when it comes back in the same family, or in neighbors.

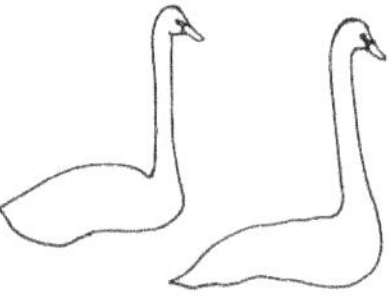

The departed soul retains the memory of its past experiences only in their essence, not in their form of detail. It is only if the soul brings back some past personality or personalities as part of its present manifestation that it is likely to remember the details of the past life. Otherwise, it is only by Yogadrishti that the memory comes.

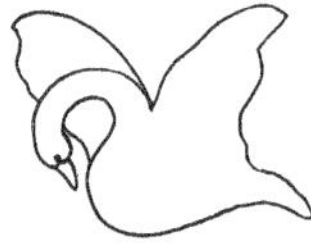

I have told you many times and I could not repeat it too often, that one is not built up of one single piece. We have within us many states of being and each state of being has its own life. All this is put together in one single body, so long as you have a body, and acts through that single body; so that gives you the feeling that it is one single person, a single being. But there are many beings and particularly there are concentrations on different levels: just as you have a physical being, you have a vital being, you have a mental being, you have a psychic being, you have many others and all possible intermediaries. But it is a little complicated, you might not understand.

Suppose you were living a life of desire, passion and impulse: you live with your vital being dominant in you; but if you live with spiritual effort, with great good will, the desire to do things well and an unselfishness, a will for progress, you live with the psychic being dominant in you. Then, when you are about to leave your body, all these beings start to disperse. Only if you are a very advanced yogi and have been able to unify your being around the divine centre, do these beings remain bound together. If you have not known how to unify yourself, then at the time of death all that is dispersed: each one returns to its domain. For example, with regard to the vital being, all your different desires will be separated and each one run towards its own realisation, quite independently, for the physical being will no longer be there to hold them together. But if you have united your consciousness with the psychic consciousness, when you die you remain conscious of your psychic being and the psychic being returns to the psychic world which is a world of bliss and delight and peace and tranquillity and of a growing knowledge. So, if you like to call that a paradise, it is all right; because in fact, to the extent to which you are identified with your psychic being, you remain conscious of it, you are one with it, and it is immortal and goes to its immortal domain to enjoy a perfectly happy life or rest. If you like to call that paradise, call it paradise. If you are good, if you have become conscious of your psychic and live in it, well, when your body dies, you will go with your psychic being to take rest in the psychic world, in a blissful state.

But if you have lived in your vital with all its impulses, each impulse will try to realise itself here and there... For example, a miser who is concentrated upon his money, when he dies, the part of the vital that was interested in his money will be stuck there and will continue to watch over the money so that nobody may take it. ... Now, if you live exclusively in your physical consciousness (it is difficult, for you have, after all, thoughts and feelings, but if you live exclusively in your physical), when the physical being disappears, you disappear at the same time, it is finished.... There is a spirit of the form: your form has a spirit which persists for seven days after your death. The doctors have declared that you are dead, but the spirit of your form lives, and not only does it live but it is conscious in most of the cases. But that lasts for seven or eight days and afterwards it is dissolved. I am not speaking of yogis; I am speaking of ordinary people. Yogis have no laws, it is quite different; for them the world is different. I am speaking to you of ordinary men living an ordinary life; for these it is like that.

So the conclusion is that if you want to preserve your consciousness, it would be better to centralise it on a part of your being that is immortal; otherwise it will vanish like a flame in the air. And it is very fortunate, for if it were otherwise, there would be perhaps gods or types of superior men who would create hells and heavens as they do in their material imagination, where they would imprison you; you would be imprisoned in heaven or in hell according as you pleased or displeased them. It would be a very critical situation and happily it is not like that.

Sometimes when people are dying, they know they are about to die. Why don't they tell the spirit [of death] to go away?

Ah! Well, that depends upon the people. Two things are necessary. First of all, nothing in your being, no part of your being should want to die. That does not happen often. You have always a defeatist in you somewhere: something that is tired, something that is disgusted, something that has had enough of it, something that is lazy, something that does not want to struggle and says: "Well! Ah! Let it be finished, so much the better." That is sufficient, you are dead.

But it is a fact: if nothing, absolutely nothing in you consents to die, you will not die. For someone to die, there is always a second, perhaps the hundredth part of a second, when he gives his consent. If there is not this second of consent, he does not die.

I knew people who should have really died according to all physical and vital laws; and they refused. They said: "No, I will not die", and they lived. There are others who do not need at all to die, but they are of that kind and say: "Ah! Well! Yes, so much the better, it will be finished," and it is finished. Even that much, even nothing more than that: you need not have a persistent wish, you have only to say: "Well, yes, I have had enough!" and it is finished. So it is truly like that. As you say, you may have death standing by your bedside and tell him: "I do not want you, go away", and it will be obliged to go away. But usually one gives way, for one must struggle, one must be strong, one must be very courageous and enduring, must have a great faith in the necessity of life; like someone, for example, who feels very strongly that he has still something to do and he must absolutely do it. But who is sure he has not within him the least bit of a defeatist, somewhere, who just yields and says: "It is all right"?... It is here, the necessity of unifying oneself.

Whatever the way we follow, the subject we study, we always arrive at the same result. The most important thing for an individual is to unify himself around his divine centre; in that way he becomes a true individual, master of himself and his destiny. Otherwise, he is a plaything of forces that toss him about like a piece of cork on a river. He goes where he does not want to go, he is made to do things he does not want to do, and finally he loses himself in a hole without having any strength to recover. But if you are consciously organised, unified around the divine centre, ruled and directed by it, you are master of your destiny. That is worth the trouble of attempting.... In any case, I find it preferable to be the master rather than the slave. It is a rather unpleasant sensation to feel yourself pulled by the strings and made to do things whether you want to or not — that is quite irrelevant — but to be compelled to act because something pulls you by the strings, something which you do not even see — that is exasperating. However, I do not know, but I found it very exasperating, even when I was quite a child. At five, it began to seem to me quite intolerable and I sought for a way so that it might be otherwise — without people getting a chance to scold me. For I knew nobody who could help me and I did not have the chance that you have, someone who can tell you: "This is what you have to do!" There was nobody to tell me that. I had to find it out all by myself. And I found it. I started at five. And you, you were five long ago....*Voilà.*

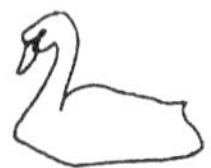

The psychic being's choice at the time of death does not *work out* the next formation of the personality, it *fixes* it. When it enters the psychic world, it begins to assimilate the essence of its experience and by that assimilation is formed the future psychic personality in accordance with the fixation already made. When this assimilation is over, it is ready for a new birth; but the less developed beings do not work out the whole thing for themselves, there are beings and forces of the higher world who have this work. Also, when it comes to birth, it is not sure the forces of the physical world will not come across the working out of what it wanted – its own new instrumentation may not be strong enough for that purpose; for, there is the interaction of its own energies and the cosmic forces here. There may be frustration, division, a partial working out – many things may happen. All that is not a rigid machinery, it is the working out of complex forces.

It may be added, however, that a developed psychic being is much more conscious in this transition and works out much of it itself. The time depends also on the development and on a certain rhythm of the being – for some there is practically immediate rebirth, for others it takes longer, but for some it may take centuries; but here, again, once the psychic being is sufficiently developed, it is free to choose its own rhythm and its own intervals.

The ordinary theories are too mechanical – and that is the case also with the idea of *punya* and *papa* [punishment and reward] and their results in the next life. There are certainly results of the energies put forth in a past life, but not on that rather infantile principle. A good man's suffering in this life would be a proof, according to the orthodox theory, that he had been a very great villain in his past life. A bad man's prospering would be a proof that he had been quite angelic in his last visit to earth and sown a large crop of virtues and meritorious actions to reap this bumper crop of good fortune. Too symmetrical to be true.

The object of birth being growth by experience, whatever reactions come to past deeds must be for the being to learn and grow, not as lollipops for good boys in the class (in the past), and canings for the bad ones. The real sanction of good and ill is not good fortune for the one and bad fortune for the other, but this; that good leads us towards a higher nature which is eventually lifted above suffering, and it pulls us towards the lower nature which remains always in the circle of suffering and evil.

As one drawn by the grandeur of the Void
The soul attracted leaned to the Abyss:
It longed for the adventure of Ignorance
And the marvel and surprise of the Unknown
And the endless possibility that lurked
In the womb of Chaos and in Nothing's gulf
Or looked from the unfathomed eyes of Chance.
It tired of its unchanging happiness,
It turned away from immortality:
It was drawn to hazard's call and danger's charm,
It yearned to the pathos of grief, the drama of pain,
Perdition's peril, the wounded bare escape,
The music of ruin and its glamour and crash,
The savour of pity and the gamble of love
And passion and the ambiguous face of Fate.

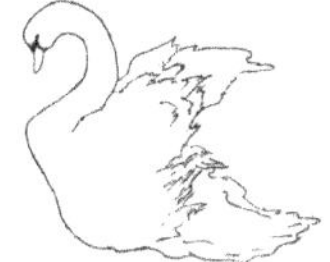

*Can it happen that the psychic being does not fall at the place
where it wanted to take birth?*

If a psychic being sees from its psychic world a light on the earth,
it may rush down there without knowing exactly where it is.
Everything is possible. But if the psychic being is very conscious,
sufficiently conscious, it will seek the light of aspiration in a
precise place, because of the culture, the education it will find
there. This happens much more frequently than one believes,
especially in somewhat educated circles. An intelligent woman
with some artistic or philosophical culture, a beginning of
conscious individuality, may aspire that the child she is going to
have may be the best possible according to her idea or according
to what she has read. Hence it is not so very complicated to
find a place. The number of psychic beings born constantly
being considerable, if each time exceptional conditions have
to be found it would be difficult. Surely, there are instances
where the psychic being seems to have fallen headlong and
been stunned, but this is bad luck; in such a case it generally

requires a long time to wake up. It is bad luck in the sense that it probably lacked a certain power of discrimination, or perhaps it had to face certain forces which thwarted its decision and won a partial victory over it. There are a thousand possibilities, you know. One cannot say that everything goes according to the same plan — every psychic being is different. 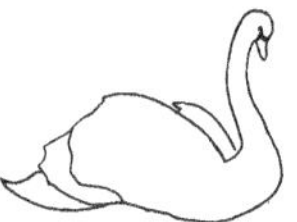

Once in the immortal boundlessness of Self,
In a vast of Truth and Consciousness and Light
The soul looked out from its felicity.
It felt the Spirit's interminable bliss,
It knew itself deathless, timeless, spaceless, one,
It saw the Eternal, lived in the Infinite.
Then, curious of a shadow thrown by Truth,
It strained towards some otherness of self,
It was drawn to an unknown Face peering through night.
It sensed a negative infinity,
A void supernal whose immense excess
Imitating God and everlasting Time
Offered a ground for Nature's adverse birth
And Matter's rigid hard unconsciousness
Harbouring the brilliance of a transient soul
That lights up birth and death and ignorant life.

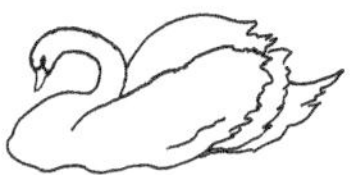

For past lives, are there any general rules, broad outlines, or is everything possible?

All depends on the category to which one belongs, and the degree of the psychic being's development. If the psychic being is in an advanced stage, near maturity, the choice before death... is quite real and this choice means that everything is possible; but in other cases, the rebirth takes place almost automatically. The will of the psychic being is not developed and it does not choose. Hence, there are no rules. It depends very much on circumstances, and especially on the line of formation which the psychic being will follow, and that depends on its origin. It is difficult to say in the matter of sex, that may vary for a long time. As the consciousness grows and gains some unity of action, of consciousness, it can choose to follow one line to the exclusion of another, but before this choice, through innumerable creations, you have been undoubtedly of different sexes. That is why perhaps some women have a masculine character, and visa versa, or have tendencies opposite to their own sex. But at the time of the "choice" one may decide to belong to the creatrix Consciousness or to the immobile Witness. That depends upon the origin.

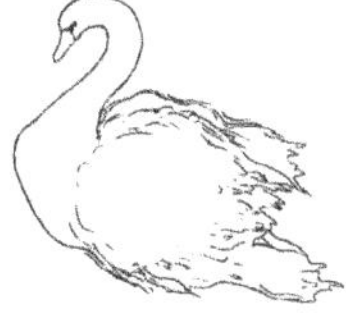

(The Mother listens to a letter of Sri Aurobindo.)

(Question:) X asked me if in the course of rebirths a woman can become a man, and a man a woman. He thought of certain feminine traits in him that could be explained thus. I would also like to know if there is in the psychic being itself something like sex?

(Answer:) Not sex exactly, but what might be called the masculine and feminine principle. It is a difficult question [whether sex is altered in rebirth]. There are certain lines the reincarnation follows and so far as my experience goes and general experience goes, one follows usually a single line. But the alteration of sex cannot be declared impossible. There may be some who do alternate. The presence of feminine traits in a male does not necessarily indicate a past feminine birth - they may come in the general play of forces and their formations. There are besides qualities common to both sexes. Also a fragment of the psychological personality may have been associated with a birth not ones own. One can say of a certain person of the past, "that was not myself, but a fragment of my psychological

personality was present in him." Rebirth is a complex affair and not so simple in its mechanism as in the popular idea.
He says it's "fragments"?

Yes, that there may be fragments.

It must be correct, it fits with my own experience.

The psychic, that's true, has masculine and feminine tendencies, but it's not "man" or "woman": the psychic is sexless.

And as he says, it's quite a complex affair; there are all possibilities. There's nothing one can declare to be impossible. ✸

You know, the story of the "soul leaving the body," what childishness! Because I had that experience, too, of leaving (not the soul! It's entirely independent, always and in everyone), of leaving the psychic being, the individual psychic being. When I went away from here in 1915, I left my psychic being here deliberately. I left it here, I didn't take it with me. So the body can live without psychic being (it was rather sick, by the way, but that wasn't the reason - it's again the taste for drama! ... Oh, always the taste for drama!).

It's more difficult to live without the psychic being, on the other hand. The psychic being, of course, is the clothing - the individualized clothing - between the eternal soul and the transitory body; and [from life to life] it grows more formed, individualized, more and more individually conscious. When that leaves the body, the rest generally follows. But I had the experience of doing it deliberately, so I KNOW. One has to know how to do it, but it can be done. My psychic being stayed here with Sri Aurobindo, and I left with my mental, vital and physical beings. It was a ... slightly precarious condition. But as I also kept the contact quite consciously, it could be done. ✸

Communications from the psychic do not come in a mental form. They are not ideas or reasonings. They have their own character quite distinct from the mind, something like a feeling that comprehends itself and acts.

By its very nature, the psychic is calm, quiet and luminous, understanding and generous, wide and progressive. Its constant effort is to understand and progress.

The mind describes and explains.

The psychic sees and understands. 

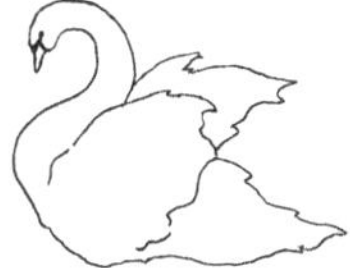

One may have knowledge from the psychic — though it is of another kind and is not formulated as in the mind. It is a sort of inner certitude which makes you do the right thing at the right moment and in the right way, without necessarily passing through the reason or mental formation.

For instance, one may act with a perfect knowledge of what should be done, and without intervention — the least intervention --- of the reasoning mind. The mind is silent. It simply looks on and listens in order to register things, it does not act. 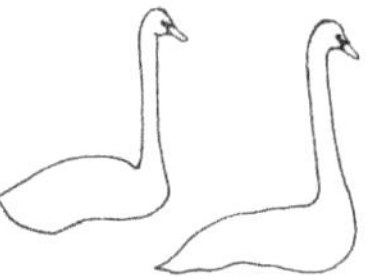

Once the psychic has come to the front, can it withdraw again?

Yes. Generally one has a series of experiences of identification, very intense at first, which later gradually diminish, and then one day you find that they have disappeared. Still you must not be disturbed, for it is quite a common phenomenon. But next time — the second time — the contact is more easily obtained. And then comes a moment, which is not very far off, when as soon as one concentrates and aspires, one gets a contact. One may not have the power of keeping it all the time, but can get it at will. Then, from that moment things become very easy. When one feels a difficulty or there is a problem to be solved, when one wants to make progress or there is just a depression to conquer or an obstacle to be overcome or else simply for the joy of identification (for it is an experience that gives a very concrete joy; at the moment of identification one truly feels a very, very great joy), then, at any moment whatever, one may pause, concentrate for a while and aspire, and quite naturally the contact is established and problems which were to be solved are solved. Simply to concentrate — to sit down and concentrate — to aspire in this way, and the contact is made, so to say, instantaneously.

There comes a time, as I said, when this does not leave you, that is, it is in the depths of the consciousness and supports all that you do, and you never lose the contact. Then many things disappear. For instance, depression is one of these things, discontentment, revolt, fatigue, depression, all these difficulties. And if one makes it a habit to step back, as we say, in one's consciousness and see on the screen of one's psychic consciousness — see all the circumstances, all the events, all the ideas, all the knowledge, everything — at that moment one sees that and has an altogether sure guide for everything that one may do. But this, perforce, takes a very long time to come.

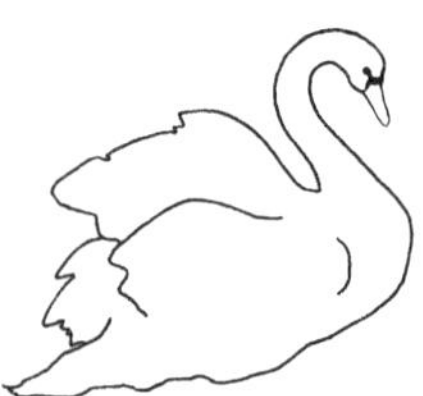

Onward they journeyed through the drifting ways
Vaguely companioned by the glimmering mists.
But faster now all fled as if perturbed
Escaping from the clearness of her soul.
A heaven-bird upon jewelled wings of wind
Bourne like a coloured and embosomed fire,
By spirits carried in a pearl-hued cave,
On through the enchanted dimness moved her soul. 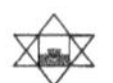

It depends on the emotion and it also depends on what you call an emotion. For example, there is a state where, if you find yourself in the presence of a very precise, very clear psychic movement, a distinctly psychic movement — this happens quite often — the emotion is so powerful that tears come to your eyes. You are not sad, you are not happy, neither one nor the other; it doesn't correspond to any particular feeling, but it is an intensity of emotion which comes from something that is clearly, precisely psychic. It may be in yourself, but it is even more often in someone else. When you are in contact with an act, a movement, a manifestation which belongs to the psychic, then, all of a sudden, the eyes are filled with tears. If you call that an emotion... obviously it is an emotion. But usually, it comes from one thing: the physical being has a not very conscious but very intense longing for a contact with the psychic life. It feels poor, destitute, isolated and abandoned when it is not in contact with the psychic being. Not one physical being in a million is aware of this. But this kind of impression of being lost, left hanging, without protection, without support, of lacking something and not knowing what it is, something you don't understand but which you lack, an emptiness somewhere: well, this comes more often than one thinks — people have no idea what it is. But then, when for some reason or other this consciousness suddenly comes into contact with a clearly psychic phenomenon, with psychic forces, psychic vibrations, the feeling is so strong, so strong that certainly, most often, the body can hardly hold it. It is like a joy that is too great, that overflows on all sides, that you can't contain, can't hold in yourself. It is like that. There is suddenly a sort of revelation, not very conscious, not clearly expressed, the revelation of... this is it, this is what I must have. And it is so powerful, so powerful that it gives you an emotion, which is made up of so many things that you can hardly say what it is. These are emotions that are not vital.

Vital emotions are of an altogether different nature — they are very clear, very precise, you can express them very distinctly; they are violent, they usually fill you with an intensity, a restlessness, sometimes a great satisfaction. And then the opposite comes with the same force. And so people, many people think — we have mentioned this several times already — some people imagine they experience love only when it is like that, when love is in the vital, when it comes with all the movements of the vital, all this intensity, this, violence, this precision, this glamour, this brightness. And when that is absent they say, "Oh, this is not love."

And yet that is exactly how love gets distorted: already it is no longer love, it is beginning to be passion. And this is an almost universal error among human beings.

Some people are full of a very pure, very high, very selfless psychic love and yet they know nothing about it and think they are cold, dry and without love because this admixture of vital vibration is absent. For them love begins and ends with this vibration.

And as it is something highly unstable which has movements and reactions and violences of all kinds, in depression as in satisfaction, love is something very ephemeral for these people: they have minutes of love in their lives. It may last a few hours and then it becomes dull and flat again and they imagine that love has deserted them. As I said, some people are quite beyond that, they have been able to control it in such a way that it does not get mixed up with anything else; they have in themselves this psychic love which is full of self-forgetfulness, of self-giving, compassion, generosity, nobility of life, and is a great power of identification. So most of these people think they are cold or indifferent — they are very nice people, you see, but they do not love — and sometimes they themselves do not know. I have known people who thought they had no love because they didn't have this vital vibration. Usually, when people speak of emotions, they are speaking of vital emotions. But there is another kind of emotion which is of an infinitely higher order and doesn't express itself in the same way, which has just as much intensity, but an intensity that is under control, contained, condensed, concentrated, and is an extraordinary dynamic power.

True love can achieve extraordinary things, but it is rare. All kinds of miracles can be done out of love for the person one loves — not for everyone, but for the people or the person one loves. But it has to be a love free from all vital mixture, an absolutely pure and selfless love which demands nothing in return, which expects nothing in return.

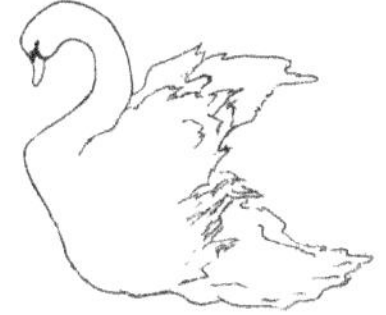

FLAME-WIND

A flame-wind ran from the gold of the East,
Leaped on my soul with the breath of a seven-fold noon.
Wings of the angel, gallop of the beast!
Mind and body on fore, but the heart in swoon.

O flame, thou bringest he strength of the noon,
But where are the voices of morn and the stillness of eve?
Where the pale-blue wine of the moon?
Mind and life are in flower, but the heart must grieve.

Gold in the mind and the life-flame's red
Make of the heavens a splendour, the earth a blaze,
But the white and rose of the heart are dead.
Flame-wind pass! I will wait for love in the silent ways.

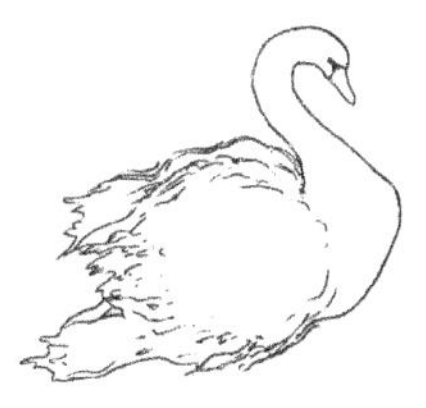

It is also a mistake to think that the vital alone has warmth and the psychic is something frigid without any flame in it. A clear limpid goodwill is a very good and desirable thing. But that is not what is meant by psychic love. Love is love and not merely goodwill. Psychic love can have a warmth and a flame as intense and more intense than the vital, only it is a pure fire, not dependent on the satisfaction of ego-desire or on the eating up of the fuel it embraces. It is a white flame, not a red one; but white heat is not inferior to the red variety in its ardour. It is true that the psychic love does not usually get its full play in human relations and human nature; it finds the fullness of its fire and ecstasy more easily when it is lifted towards the Divine. In the human relation the psychic love gets mixed up with other elements which seek at once to use it and overshadow it. It gets an outlet for its own full intensities only at rare moments. Otherwise it comes in only as an element, but even so it contributes all the higher things in a love fundamentally vital — all the finer sweetness, tenderness, fidelity, self-giving, self-sacrifice, reachings of soul to soul, idealising sublimations that lift up human love beyond itself, come from the psychic. If it could dominate and govern and transmute the other elements, mental, vital, physical, of human love, then love could be on the earth some reflection or preparation of the real thing, an integral union of the soul and its instruments in a dual life. But even some imperfect appearance of that is rare.

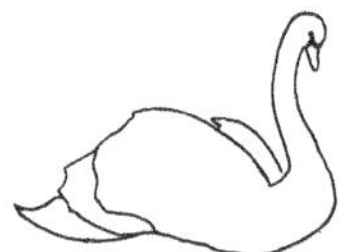

So she fared on across her silent self.
To a road she came thronged with an ardent crowd
Who sped brilliant, fire-footed, sunlight-eyed,
Pressing to reach the world's mysterious wall,
And pass through masked doorways into outer mind
Where the Light comes not nor the mystic voice,
Messengers from our subliminal greatnesses,
Guests from the cavern of the secret soul.
Into dim spiritual somnolence they break
Or shed wide wonder on our waking self,
Ideas that haunt us with their radiant tread,
Dreams that are hints of unborn Reality,
Strange goddesses with deep-pooled magical eyes,
Strong wind-haired gods carrying the harps of hope,
Great moon-hued visions gliding through gold air,
Aspiration's sun-dream head and star-carved limbs,
Emotions making common hearts sublime. …

"O Savitri, from thy hidden soul we come.
We are the messengers, the occult gods
Who help men's drab and heavy ignorant lives
To wake to beauty and the wonder of things
Touching them with glory and divinity;
In evil we light the deathless flame of good
And hold the torch of knowledge on ignorant roads;
We are thy will and all men's will towards Light.
O human copy and disguise of God
Who seekst the deity thou keepest hid
And livest by the Truth thou hast not known,
Follow the world's winding highway to its source.
There in the silence few have ever reached,
Thou shalt see the Fire burning on the bare stone
And the deep cavern of thy secret soul.

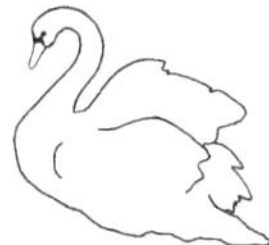

How can one know that the psychic being is in front?

My child. when it happens, one understands. It is exactly so long as one doesn't understand that it means that it hasn't come. This is like people asking you. "How can I know whether I am in contact with the Divine?" That itself is enough to prove that they are not. For if they are they can no longer ask the question. It is something understood. For the psychic it is the same thing. When the psychic is in front one knows it, and there is no possibility of any doubt. Consequently one no longer asks the question.

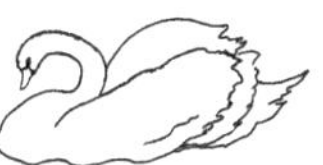

Even now hints of a luminous Truth like stars
Arise in the mind-mooned splendour of Ignorance;
Even now the deathless Lover's touch we feel:
If the chamber door is even a little ajar,
What then can hinder God from stealing in
Or forbid his kiss on the sleeping soul?

In the 'Questions and Answers' you speak of the 'reversal of consciousness.' Is this synonymous with the psychic realization? Because in one Conversation you connect the two things: the reversal of consciousness and the discovery of the psychic being.

It's the result of this discovery. In fact, it's the result of union with the psychic being. 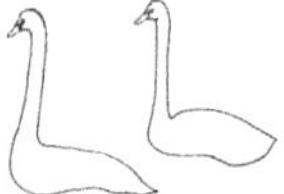

Then Savitri following the great winding road
Came where it dwindled into a narrow path
Trod only by rare wounded pilgrim feet.
A few bright forms emerged from unknown depths
And looked at her with calm immortal eyes.
There was no sound to break the brooding hush;
One felt the silent nearness of the soul.

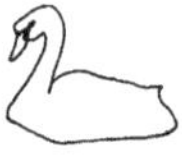

THE SELF'S INFINITY

I have become what before Time I was.
   A secret hush has quieted thought and sense:
All things by the agent Mind created pass
   Into a void and mute magnificence.

My life is a silence grasped by timeless hands;
   The world is drowned in an immortal gaze,
Naked my spirit from its vestures stands;
   I am alone with my own self for space.

My heart is a centre of infinity,
   My body a dot in the soul's vast expanse.
All being's huge abyss wakes under me,
   Once screened in a gigantic Ignorance.

A momentless immensity pure and bare,
I stretch to an eternal everywhere.

These last few days I've had a series of experiences on this very subject, very interesting experiences.... With the same person, whom I see every day, let's say, or very often, the impression the contact has (an impression that stays on for a shorter or longer time) depends on the presence of the psychic. With the same person, you understand, the same relationship, at certain times it becomes full and you have the sense of something ... yes, full - not exactly "living," but ... (I can't say "solid" because there's nothing hard about it), but full, substantial; then, at other times, it's thin, fleeting, neutral. And I have observed (with the same people in the same circumstances), at times you have the sense of a ... more than living contact (the word "living" isn't enough), an EXISTENT contact, rather; an existent, durable contact (but not "durable" in time: durable in its nature); at other times with the very same people (often in the same circumstances), it's thin, flat, it's dry, superficial - it may be very active, apparently very living, but it has no depth.... And I have seen that it is when the psychic participates and when it doesn't.

So I have now reached the point where every minute I can feel ("feel," I don't mean perceive psychically, I mean feel materially) when the psychic is there and when it isn't. It's very interesting. These last few days. ✿

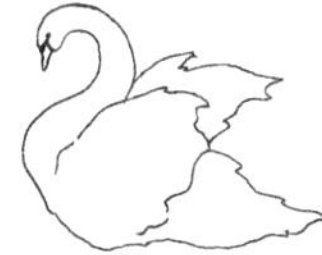

In order to find the soul you must go in this way (gesture of going deep within), like this, draw back from the surface, withdraw deep within and enter, enter, enter, go down, down, down into a very deep hole, silent, immobile, and there, there's a kind of... something warm, quiet, rich in substance and very still, and very full, like a sweetness — that is the soul.

And if one is insistent and is conscious oneself, then there comes a kind of plenitude which gives the feeling of something complete that contains unfathomable depths in which, should one enter, one feels that many secrets would be revealed... like the reflection in very peaceful waters of something that is eternal. And one no longer feels limited by time.

One has the feeling of having always been and of being for eternity.

That is when one has touched the core of the soul.

And if the contact has been conscious and complete enough, it liberates you from the bondage of outer form; you no longer feel that you live only because you have a body. That is usually the ordinary sensation of the being, to be so tied to this outer form that when one thinks of "myself' one thinks of the body. That is the usual thing. The personal reality is the body's reality. It is only when one has made an effort for inner development and tried to find something that is a little more stable in one's being, that one can begin to feel that this "something" which is permanently conscious throughout all ages and all change, this something must be "myself'. But that already requires a study that is rather deep. Otherwise if you think "I am going to do this", "I need that", it is always your body, a small kind of will which is a mixture of sensations, of more or less confused sentimental reactions, and still more confused thoughts which form a mixture and are animated by an impulse, an attraction, a desire, some sort of a will; and all that momentarily becomes "myself" — but not directly, for one does not conceive this "myself" as independent of the head, the trunk, the arms and legs and all that moves — it is very closely linked.

It is only after having thought much, seen much, studied much, observed much that you begin to realise that the one is more or less independent of the other and that the will behind can make it either act or not act, and you begin not to be completely identified with the movement, the action, the realisation — that something is floating. But you have to observe much to see that.

And then you must observe much more still to see that this, the second thing that is there, this kind of active conscious will, is set in motion by "something else" which watches, judges, decides and tries to found its decisions on knowledge — that happens even much later. And so, when you begin to see this "something else", you begin to see that it has the power to set in motion the second thing, which is an active will; and not only that, but that it has a very direct and very important action on the reactions, the feelings, the sensations, and that finally it can have control over all the movements of the being—this part which watches, observes, judges and decides.

That is the beginning of control.

When one becomes conscious of that, one has seized the thread, and when one speaks of control, one can know, "Ah! yes, this is what has the power of control."

This is how one learns to look at oneself.   

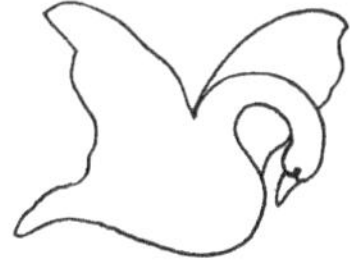

A house was there all made of flame and light
And crossing a wall of doorless living fire
There suddenly she met her secret soul.
A being stood immortal in transience,
Deathless dallying with momentary things,
In whose wide eyes of tranquil happiness
Which pity and sorrow could not abrogate
Infinity turned its gaze on finite shapes:
Observer of the silent steps of the hours,
Eternity upheld the minute's acts
And the passing scenes of the Everlasting's play.
In the mystery of its selecting will,
In the Divine Comedy a participant,
The Spirit's conscious representative,
God's delegate in our humanity,
Comrade of the universe, the Transcendent's ray,
She had come into the mortal body's room
To play at ball with Time and Circumstance.
A joy in the world her master movement here,
The passion of the game lighted her eyes:
A smile on her lips welcomed earth's bliss and grief,
A laugh was her return to pleasure and pain.
All things she saw as a masquerade of Truth
Disguised in the costumes of Ignorance,
Crossing the years to immortality;
All she could front with the strong spirit's peace.

Identified with the mind and body and life,
It takes on itself their anguish and defeat,
Bleeds with Fate's whips and hangs upon the cross,
Yet is the unwounded and immortal self
Supporting the actor in the human scene.
Through this she sends us her glory and her powers,
Pushes to wisdom's heights, through misery's gulfs;
She gives us strength to do our daily task
And sympathy that partakes of others' grief
And the little strength we have to help our race,
We who must fill the role of the universe
Acting itself out in a slight human shape
And on our shoulders carry the struggling world.
This is in us the godhead small and marred;
In this human portion of divinity
She seats the greatness of the Soul in Time
To uplift from light to light, from power to power,
Till on a heavenly peak it stands, a king.
In body weak, in its heart an invincible might,
It climbs stumbling, held up by an unseen hand,
A toiling spirit in a mortal shape.
Here in this chamber of flame and light they met;
They looked upon each other, knew themselves,
The secret deity and its human part,
The calm immortal and the struggling soul.
Then with a magic transformation's speed
They rushed into each other and grew one.

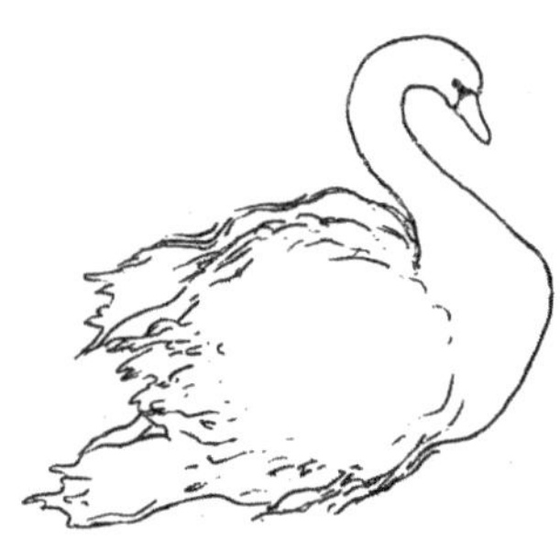

THE BODY

This body which was once my universe,
    Is now a pittance carried by the soul, -
Its Titan's motion bears this scanty purse,
    Pacing through vastness to a vaster goal.

Too small it was to meet the giant need
    That only infinitude can satisfy:
He keeps it still, for in its folds is hid
    His secret passport to eternity.

In his front an endless Time and Space deploy
    The landscape of their golden happenings;
His heart is filled with sweet and violent joy,
    His mind is upon great and distant things.

How grown with all the world coterminous
Is the little dweller in this narrow house!

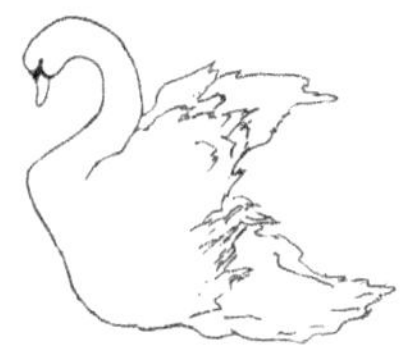

A channel of the mighty Mother's choice,
The immortal's will took into its calm control
Our blind or erring government of life;
A loose republic once of wants and needs,
Then bowed to the uncertain sovereign mind,
Life now obeyed to a diviner rule
And every act became an act of God.
In the kingdom of the lotus of the heart
Love chanting its pure hymeneal hymn
Made life and body mirrors of sacred joy
And all the emotions gave themselves to God.
In the navel lotus' broad imperial range
Its proud ambitions and its master lusts
Were tamed into instruments of a great calm sway
To do a work of God on earthly soil.

But she is sweet, your mother.... She is going to have the joy of her soul. You know, there is a joy in being more conscious of one's soul than of the material world - you may keep yourself busy, you may see clearly, you may understand, you may do what you have to do, all that remains, it's very fine, but, behind, there is ... a Light. A light, something warm, warm with a luminous, golden warmth. It's really the sense of immortality, of something that doesn't depend on a form or on circumstances. It's a consciousness in which one instantly has the feeling that there was no beginning, there is no end.... And a sort of very strong sweetness, very strong, behind everything. It takes you through life; even all the difficulties don't matter when you have caught hold of that. It's something very intimate, which expresses itself with difficulty, but which is like a support, something that holds you up always, in any circumstances.

That's what your mother will have.

She must be living it, maybe unknowingly; she must already have it a little, a beginning.

But when one has it consciously, then…then, in reality, circumstances don't matter much.

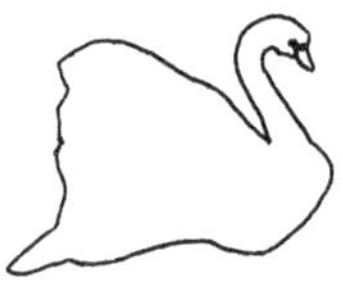

It was 11:00 A.M. (I think he died at 9:30 A.M.). I go there (I don't remember if it was in the morning or early in the afternoon, anyhow it was very soon after his death), I sit down, the son is ushered in, and along with him comes a small boy, no taller than this *(gesture)*, all golden, joyous, alive, happy! ... And he rushed to me. He stayed like that, leaning against me, quite still. And how he laughed! How happy he was!

It was M., his psychic being.

Ever so lovely! All luminous - luminous with a golden light - and so happy, so glad! Like a baby, no bigger than this *(gesture)*. Waving his arms and legs about, so happy! He stayed there - stayed put. So naturally, I received him and did the needful.

I've seen thousands of cases, you know, but it's the first time I've seen that! And he had a remarkable knowledge, because in order not to risk any hitch, he clung to his son and urged him to come to me so as to make sure of reaching me without mishap, without any interference from the adverse forces, from currents and all sorts of things. He clung to his son, who was quite unaware of it, except that something in him WANTED him to come to me. And the poor son was crying; I told him, "Don't worry, he is very happy"! *(Mother laughs)*

And lovely! A lovely thing. The sight of it filled me with joy - so happy, so happy, he seemed to be saying, "At last I am with you! I won't budge now, no one can take me away." This small.

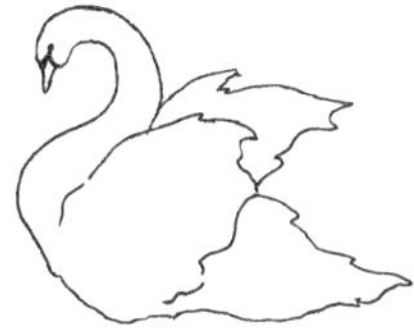

THE DIVINE WORKER

I face earth's happenings with an equal soul;
    In all are heard Thy steps, Thy unseen feet
Tread Destiny's pathways in my front. Life's whole
    Tremendous theorem is Thou complete.

No danger can perturb my spirit's calm:
    My acts are Thine; I do Thy works and pass;
Failure is cradled on Thy deathless arm,
    Victory is Thy passage mirrored in Fortune's glass.

In this rude combat with the fate of man
    Thy smile within my heart makes all my strength;
Thy force in me labours at its grandiose plan,
    Indifferent to the Time-snake's crawling length.

No power can slay my soul; it lives in Thee.
Thy presence is my immortality.

The sense of release as if from jail always accompanies the emergence of the psychic being or the realisation of the self above. It is therefore spoken of as a liberation, *mukti*. It is a release into peace, happiness, the soul's freedom not tied down by the thousand ties and cares of the outward ignorant existence. 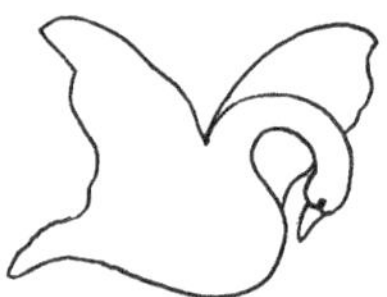

I had an experience which I found interesting, because it was the first time. It was yesterday or the day before (I forget), [Rijuta, an American disciple]. was here, just in front of me, kneeling, and I saw her psychic being towering above by this much *(gesture about eight inches)*, taller. It's the first time. Her physical being was short, and the psychic being was tall, like this. And it was a sexless being: neither man nor woman. So I said to myself (it may be always that way, I don't know, but at that time I noticed it very clearly), I said to myself, "But the psychic being is the one that will materialize and become the supramental being!"

I saw it, it was like that. There were distinctive features, but not very pronounced, and it was clearly a being that was neither male nor female, that had features of both combined. And it was taller than her, it exceeded her on every side by about this much *(gesture extending beyond the physical being by about eight inches)*. She was here, and it was like this *(gesture)*. Its color was ... this color that, if it became very material, would be Auroville's color [orange]. It was softer, as if behind a veil, it wasn't absolutely precise, but it was this color. And there was hair, but ... it was something else.

Another time maybe I'll see better.

But I found it very interesting, because that being seemed to tell me, "You're wondering what the supramental being will be - here it is! Here it is, this is it." And it was there. It was her psychic being.

Then one understands. One understands: the psychic being will materialize ... and it gives a continuity to evolution.

This creation gives you a clear impression that nothing is arbitrary, that there is a sort of divine logic behind, which isn't like our human logic, but highly superior to our logic (but it exists), and that logic was fully satisfied when I saw that.

It's odd, it was also when R. was here that I had that experience of the supramental light going through within [Mother] without causing any shadow. [See *Agenda* X of April 16 and May 3, 1969.] R. has something like that, I don't know.... And this time, it's really interesting. I was quite interested. It was there, tranquil, and saying to me, "But you're after ... well, here it is, this is it!"

So then, I understood why the mind and the vital were sent away from this body, and the psychic being was left (naturally, it was the psychic being that governed all movements earlier, so it was nothing new, but there were no more difficulties: all the complications coming from the vital and the mind, which add their imprints, their tendencies, it was all gone). So I understood: "Ah, that's it, it's this psychic being that is to become the supramental being."

I had never bothered to know what it looked like. But when I saw that, I understood. And I see it, I still see it, I have kept the memory. Its hair almost looked red, strangely (it wasn't like red hair, but it looked like it). And its expression! Such a fine expression, gently ironical ... oh, extraordinary, extraordinary!

You understand, my eyes were open, it was an almost material vision.

Then one understands! All at once, all questions vanished, it became very clear, very simple.

(silence)

And the psychic is precisely what lives on. So if it materialized, it means doing away with death. But "doing away" ... what's done away with is only what's not according to the Truth, that's what goes away - all that's incapable of being transformed in the image of the psychic, of being part of the psychic.

That's really interesting. 

When I had that experience of the psychic [with Rijuta], I said to myself, "But where is my psychic?..." It's constantly active, mingled with everything, it's what speaks; when people ask questions, I answer through it.... But I don't have the "sensation" of its presence.

I think that's when the identification is made: it's no longer a separate being, you understand.

Yes, it worried me, I wondered, "Is there something that veils?"

No! I think that's when the identification with the physical consciousness is made. Because with me it's always been like that: the minute there was union, it was over, there was no "psychic being and the rest".... What lived was the psychic. 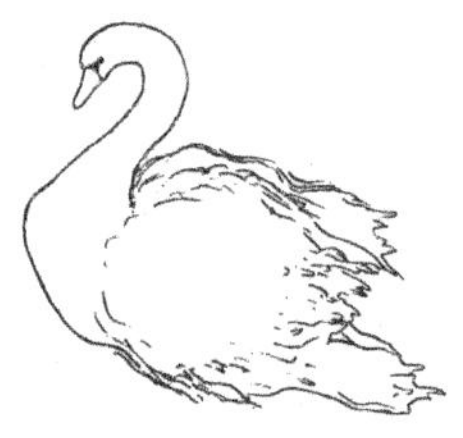

REMINISCENCE

My soul awoke at dawn and listening, heard
One voice abroad, a solitary bird,
A song not master of its note, a cry
That persevered into eternity.
My soul leaned out into the dawn to hear
In the world's solitude its winged compeer
And, harkening what the Angel had to say,
Saw luster in midnight and a secret day
Was opened to it. It beheld the stars
Born from a thought and knew how being prepares.
Then I remembered how I awoke from sleep
And made the skies, built earth, formed Ocean deep. 

In the slow process of the evolving spirit,
In the brief stade between a death and birth
A first perfection's stage is reached at last;
Out of the wood and stone of our nature's stuff
A temple is shaped where the high gods could live.
Even if the struggling world is left outside
One man's perfection still can save the world.
There is won a new proximity to the skies,
A first betrothal of the Earth to Heaven,
A deep concordat between Truth and Life:
A camp of God is pitched in human time.

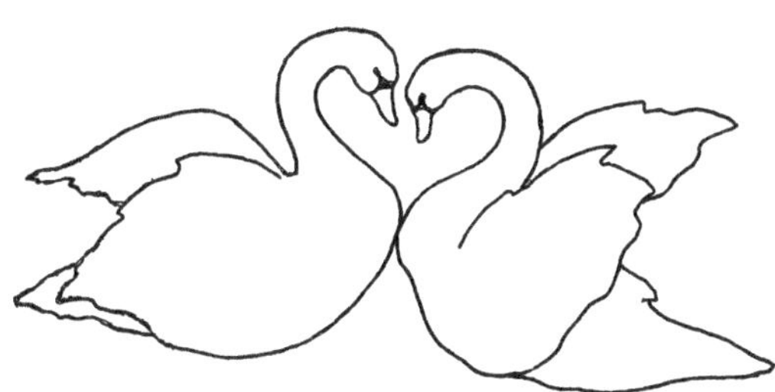

References

The passages in this book have been selected from the following publications:

Sri Aurobindo Birth Centenary library: (SABCL 5:57 = Sri Aurobindo Birth Centenary libary, Vol. 5, p. 57).

Collected Works of the Mother: (CWM 15:5 = Collected Works of the Mother, Vol. 15, p. 15).

Savitri: (Savitri, p. 499).

Mother's Agenda: (MA, 27.2.62 = Mother Agenda, February 22, 1962

The Psychic Being, a compilation publised by the Sri Aurobindo Ashram Publication Department, second edition 2008 (P.B., p. 1 = The Psychic Being, p. 1)

i	SABCL 5:570		PB, p. 182
1	SABCL 5:570	14	Savitri, p. 477
	PB, p. 8		PB, p.110
2	MA, 13.8.63		PB, p. 36
	Savitri, p. 487		PB, p. 165
	PB, p. 13	15	PB, p. 186
3	Savitri, p. 23		PB, p. 180
4	MA, 25.7.62	16	PB, p. 35
5	PB, p. 60		PB, p. 116
6	Savitri, p. 465		PB, p. 183
	PB, p 178	17	PB, p. 36
7	Savitri, p. 485		SABCL 5:47
	PB, p. 174		Savitri, p. 487
8	MA, 5.2.72	18	PB, p. 192
9	PB, p. 35	19	Savitri, p. 639
	Savitri p. 193	20	SABCL 5:143
	PB, p. 109		PB, p. 187
10	Savitri, p. 499		PB, p. 186
11	PB, p. 186	21	PB, p. 121
	MA, 25.7.62		Savitri, p. 632
12	P.B, p. 61		PB, p. 33
	PB, p. 189	22	PB, p. 43
13	PB, p. 181		PB, p. 69

24	*PB*, p. 67
	MA 9.2.72
25	*PB*, p.166
	Savitri, p. 488
	PB, p.166
	PB, p. 117
28	SABCL 5:142
	PB, p. 116
29	*PB*, p. 120
30	*PB*, p. 123
	PB, p. 116
	PB, p. 192
	PB, p. 123
32	SABCL 5:141
33	*PB*, p. 114
	MA, 5.9.62
34	*PB*, p. 123
	Savitri, p. 530
	SABCL 5:147
35	*PB*, p. 61
	PB, p. 36
	PB, p. 38
36	*Savitri* , p. 291
	PB, p. 129
37	*Savitri*, p. 293
	PB, p. 129
38	*Savitri*, p. 293
39	*PB*, p. 179
	Savitri, p. 586
	PB, p. 136
40	*Savitri*, p 292
41	*PB*, p. 155
43	*PB*, p. 151
44	MA, 29.11.67
	PB, p. 151

	CWM 5:133-38
47	*PB*, p. 138
49	*Savitri*, p. 455
	PB, p. 141
50	*Savitri*, p. 454
	PB, p. 142
51	MA, 31.10.70
52	MA, 14.6.67
53	*PB*, p. 43
	PB, p. 43
	PB, p. 115
54	*Savitri*, p. 640
55	*PB*, p. 39
57	SABCL 5:559
	PB, p. 42
58	*Savitri*, p. 500
59	*PB*, p. 114
	Savitri, p. 649
60	MA, 5.8.61
	Savitri, p. 501
	SABCL 5:142
61	MA, 19.7.67
	PB, p. 197
63	*Savitri*, p. 525
65	SABCL 5: 149
	Savitri, p. 529
66	MA, 25.12.65
	MA, 27.7.63
67	SABCL 5: 143
68	*PB*, p. 114
	M A 1.7.70
70	MA 4.7.70
	SABCL 5:41
71	*Savitri* p.531

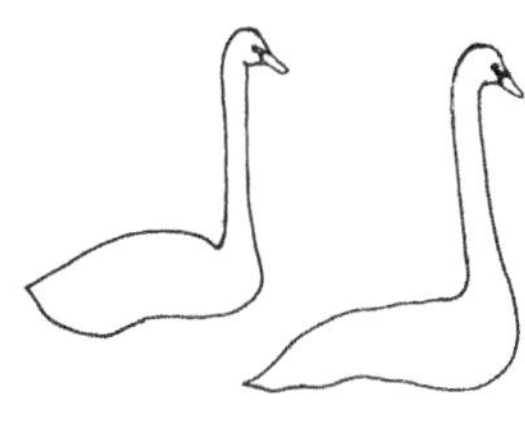

www.ingramcontent.com/pod-product-compliance
Lightning Source LLC
LaVergne TN
LVHW041228200726
843507LV00013B/2620